WITHDRAWN

DATE DUE

MAR 3 1 2009			

Demco, Inc. 38-293

Genetics
and
Hearing Loss

A Singular Audiology Textbook
Jeffrey L. Danhauer, Ph.D.
Audiology Editor

Genetics
and
Hearing Loss

Edited by

Charles I. Berlin, Ph.D.

Kenneth and Frances Barnes Bullington Professor of Hearing Science
Director, Kresge Hearing Research Laboratory of the South
Louisiana State University Health Sciences Center
Department of Otolaryngology and Biocommunication
New Orleans, Louisiana

Bronya J. B. Keats, Ph.D.

Professor and Acting Head
Department of Biometry and Genetics
Molecular and Human Genetics Center of Excellence
Louisiana State University Health Sciences Center
New Orleans, Louisiana

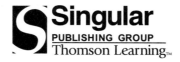

Singular
PUBLISHING GROUP
Thomson Learning™

RF 292.5 .G46x 2000

Genetics and hearing loss

Singular Publishing Group
Thomson Learning
401 West A Street, Suite 325
San Diego, California 92101-7904

Singular Publishing Group, Inc., publishes textbooks, clinical manuals, clinical reference books, journals, videos, and multimedia materials on speech-language pathology, audiology, otorhinolaryngology, special education, early childhood, aging, occupational therapy, physical therapy, rehabilitation, counseling, mental health, and voice. For your convenience, our entire catalog can be accessed on our web-site at *http//www.singpub.com.* Our mission to provide you with materials to meet the daily challenges of the everchanging health care/educational environment will remain on course if we are in touch with you. In that spirit, we welcome your feedback on our products. Please telephone (**1-800-521-8545**), fax (**1-800-774-8398**), or e-mail (*singpub@singpub.com*) your comments and requests to us.

Typeset in 10/12 Palatino by So Cal Graphics
Printed in the United States of America by RR Donnelly

Library of Congress Cataloging-in-Publication Data
Genetics and hearing loss / edited by Charles I. Berlin and Bronya Keats.
        p. ; cm. — (Singular audiology textbook)
    Includes bibliographical references and index.
    ISBN 0-7693-0103-7 (hardcover : alk. paper)
        1. Deafness—Genetic aspects—Congresses.   2. Deafness—Etiology—Congresses.   3. Ear—Abnormalities—Congresses.   I. Berlin, Charles I.   II. Keats, Bronya J. B.   III. Singular audiology text
        [DNLM: 1. Hearing Disorders—genetics—Congresses. WV 270 G32785 2000]
    RF292.5.G46 2000
    617.8'042—dc21

                                                            99-045186

Contents

Foreword

This is the fifth book in the Kresge-Mirmelstein Award cycle published and supported by Singular Publishing Group. The series was conceived by the late Rona Mirmelstein, who died in November of 1992, and Dr. Charles Berlin. Each book presents the proceedings of an annual symposium held to honor an outstanding auditory scientist, who is chosen by a consensus of peers. At the symposium, the honoree presents his or her research, and companion papers are prepared by other scientists with similar interests; all of the scientists contribute chapters to the commemorative volume, and the proceeds go to support next year's award.

This volume honors the genetic studies of Karen P. Steel, Ph.D., of the Medical Research Council's Institute of Hearing Research. Dr. Steel was selected by the previous winners of this prestigious prize to join their august ranks. The previous winners were Dr. William Brownell for his discoveries of outer hair cell motility, Dr. Robert Wenthold for his work in molecular transmitters in sensory systems, Dr. David Kemp for his discovery of otoacoustic emissions, and Dr. M. Charles Liberman for his studies of the auditory efferent system.

The symposium, entitled "Of Mice and Men: Genes, Deafness, and Otolaryngology" was held on September 27, 1998. It opened with greetings from the LSU Health Sciences Center Chancellor, Dr. Mervin L. Trail, the Dean of the Medical School, Dr. Robert L. Marier, and Otolaryngology—Head and Neck Surgery Department Head, Dr. Daniel W. Nuss, and was attended by a group of approximately 60 people. The speakers presented the results of their research in the genetics of hearing and also reviewed studies ranging from the identification and characterization of genes involved in hearing impairment to the potential for effective therapies based on knowledge of gene structure and function. Because the chapters in this book were written after the symposium, the authors have included additional information and thus the chapter titles may differ from the titles of the symposium presentation.

The first speaker at the symposium was our award winner Dr. Karen P. Steel. Her title was "A Mousey Business" and in her talk she highlighted some of the mouse studies that have advanced understanding of hereditary hearing impairment in humans. Dr. Steel's chapter title, "Of Mice and

Men (and Myosins)," reflects the important homology between the mouse and the human genomes and the usefulness of mouse models for human deafness. Her mentor, the legendary Malkeot Deol, described several of the hearing-impaired mouse strains that have facilitated research on human hearing. Dr. Steel has studied many of these mouse mutants, including *shaker-1, jerker, deafness, quivering, splotch, whirler*, and *Bronx waltzer*. These studies have been instrumental in advancing our understanding of the biological basis of hearing impairment.

Among our other distinguished speakers was Dr. Thomas Friedman, Chief of NIDCD's Laboratory of Molecular Genetics. His presentation, entitled "Identifying DFNB3" described the search for the gene responsible for deafness in members of families in Bali; the B in this symbol indicates that the mode of inheritance of the deafness in these families is autosomal recessive and DFNB3 was the third gene to be localized to a specific chromosomal region in families with this inheritance pattern. In his chapter Dr. Friedman clearly describes the relevance of parallel studies in the *shaker-2* mouse to the identification of DFNB3.

One of Dr. Friedman's collaborators, Dr. John Hinnant, an anthropologist at Michigan State University, studied the culture of the deaf inhabitants of Bali. They are born deaf and have adopted a sign language that is unique to their area. Dr. Hinnant contributed a chapter about these studies and this unique communication method. It is one of hundreds of such sign languages reported around the world, and a sample is presented in the accompanying CD-ROM prepared from Dr. Hinnant's tapes.

Since many readers of this book may not have seen either American Sign Language nor an equally valuable tool for teaching language to the deaf called Cued Speech (or Cued Language, see Fleetwood and Metzger's book, *Cued Language Structure*, Calliope Press, Silver Spring, Maryland, 1998), samples are also included on the CD-ROM. The ASL samples are provided courtesy of Ilene Miner, M.S.W., a social worker fluent in ASL who specializes in counseling with Deaf patients in general and with Usher syndrome patients in particular. She has been particularly instrumental in sensitizing us to the importance of code-switching ability in well-integrated Deaf people. The Cued Speech samples were provided by Dr. Catherine Quenin of the National Cued Speech Association. Both of these esteemed colleagues have taught us that we must never lose sight of the enormous variety of unique and successful adaptations that humans can make to a loss of auditory input. These adaptations can serve every bit as well as hearing and vocal output to convey language, literacy, and culture, and are viable strategies with their own intrinsic value.

Other speakers at the symposium were Drs. Bronya Keats, Mark Batzer, Prescott Deininger, and Richard Bobbin who each presented ongoing work in their laboratories and contributed a chapter to this book. In addition, the symposium featured posters on genetics and deafness and otoacoustic emissions by Drs. Peter Rigby, Matthew Money, Jer-Min Huang, and their collaborators, as well as related informal talks on Head and Neck Cancer and genetics by Drs. Nuss, Kluka, and Friedlander.

This entire series was made possible through the foresight and generosity of the Mirmelstein family and their friends. Sadly, Dr. Howard Mirmelstein died on October 11, 1999. The date was especially poignant, coming soon after his 80th birthday (9/14/99) and on the morning of the fifth anniversary of his wedding to Betty Mirmelstein. This book is dedicated to him and to his family who have supported our work and our clinical, scientific, and fund-raising goals for many years.

Finally, no book after 1997 in this series is complete without acknowledging the far-sighted, thoughtful and committed munificence of Frances Barnes Bullington. Mrs. Bullington, who is a retired speech pathologist, funded the Regents-supplemented Professorship which Dr. Berlin now holds, and has made a bequest to fund a Chair as well. At this time our Board of Regents accepts petitions to supplement donated funds of $600,000 so that they reach the $1 million needed to support a Chair in perpetuity. It is this generosity of purse as well as spirit, and commitment to our work, that will ultimately leave our Otolaryngology Department with both a Professorship and a Chair funded in the names of Kenneth and Frances Barnes Bullington. We will be forever indebted to her.

Charles I. Berlin, Ph.D.
Kenneth and Frances Barnes Bullington Professor of Hearing Science
Professor of Otolaryngology—Head and Neck Surgery
Director, Kresge Hearing Research Laboratory of the South

Bronya J. B. Keats, Ph.D.
Professor of Biometry and Genetics
Director, LSUHSC Molecular and Human Genetics Center of Excellence
Acting Head, Department of Biometry and Genetics

Contributors

David W. Anderson
Laboratory of Molecular Genetics
National Institute on Deafness and
    Other Communication Disorders
National Institutes of Health
Rockville, Maryland

I. Nyoman Arhya
Biochemistry and Microscopic
    Anatomy
Faculty of Medicine
Udayana University
Bali, Indonesia

James H. Asher, Jr.
Department of Zoology
Michigan State University
East Lansing, Michigan

Grace B. Athas
Department of Otoloaryngology
Tulane University Medical Center
New Orleans, Louisiana

Karen B. Avraham
Department of Human Genetics
Sackler School of Medicine
Tel Aviv University
Tel Aviv, Israel

Thomas D. Barber
Laboratory of Molecular Genetics
National Institute on Deafness and
    Other Communication Disorders
National Institutes of Health
Rockville, Maryland

Anthony P. Barnes
Neuroscience Center of Excellence

Louisiana State University Health
    Sciences Center
New Orleans, Louisiana

Mark A. Batzer
Neuroscience Center of Excellence
Departments of Pathology,
    Biometry and Genetics, and
    Biochemistry and Molecular
    Biology
Stanley S. Scott Cancer Center
    Louisiana State University
    Health Sciences Center
New Orleans, Louisiana

Richard P. Bobbin
Department of
    Otorhinolaryngology and
    Biocommunication
Kresge Hearing Research
    Laboratory of the South
Louisiana State University Health
    Sciences Center
New Orleans, Louisiana

Steve D. M. Brown
MRC Mammalian Genetics Unit
Harwell, Didcot
Oxfordshire
United Kingdom

Lauren M. Buckley
Neuroscience Center of Excellence
Department of Pathology
Louisiana State University Health
    Sciences Center
New Orleans, Louisiana

Sally A. Camper
Department of Human Genetics
University of Michigan Medical
    School
Ann Arbor, Michigan

Chu Chen
Kresge Hearing Research
    Laboratory of the South
Department of
    Otorhinolaryngology and
    Biocommunication
Neuroscience Center of
    Excellence
Louisiana State University Health
    Sciences Center
New Orleans, Louisiana

Julia L. Cook
Laboratory of Molecular
    Genetics
Alton Ochsner Medical
    Foundation
New Orleans, Louisiana

Margaret M. DeAngelis
Neuroscience Center of Excellence
Louisiana State University Health
    Sciences Center
New Orleans, Louisiana

Prescott L. Deininger
Department of Environmental
    Health Sciences
Tulane Cancer Center
Tulane Medical Center
New Orleans, Louisiana

Zhining Den
Department of Biometry and
    Genetics
Louisiana State University Health
    Sciences Center
New Orleans, Louisiana

Gregory M. Ditta
Department of Pathology
Louisiana State University Health
    Sciences Center
New Orleans, Louisiana

David Dolan
Kresge Hearing Research Institute
University of Michigan
Ann Arbor, Michigan

Chadwick J. Donaldson
Departments of Pathology,
    Biometry and Genetics
Louisiana State University Health
    Sciences Center
New Orleans, Louisiana

John P. Doucet
Molecular Genetics Section
Department of Biological Sciences
Nicholls State University
Thibodeaux, Louisiana

Stacy Drury
Department of Biometry and
    Genetics
Louisiana State University Health
    Sciences Center
New Orleans, Louisiana

Robert A. Fridell
Laboratory of Molecular Genetics
National Institute on Deafness
    and Other Communication
    Disorders
National Institutes of Health
Rockville, Maryland

Thomas B. Friedman
Chief
Laboratory of Molecular Genetics
National Institute on Deafness
    and Other Communication
    Disorders
National Institutes of Health
Rockville, Maryland

John T. Hinnant
Department of Religious Studies
Michigan State University
East Lansing, Michigan

Bronya J. B. Keats
Department of Biometry and
    Genetics
Molecular and Human Genetics
    Center

Kresge Hearing Research
  Laboratory of the South
Louisiana State University Health
  Sciences Center
New Orleans, Louisiana

Anil K. Lalwani
Laboratory of Molecular Otology
Epstein Laboratories
Department of Otolaryngology—
  Head and Neck Surgery
San Francisco, California

Christopher S. LeBlanc
Neuroscience Center of Excellence
Kresge Hearing Research
  Laboratory of the South
Department of
  Otorhinolaryngology and
  Biocommunication
Louisiana State University Health
  Sciences Center
New Orleans, Louisiana

Yong Liang
Laboratory of Molecular
  Genetics
National Institute on Deafness
  and Other Communication
  Disorders
National Institutes of Health
Rockville, Maryland

Xue-Zhong Liu
MRC Mammalian Genetics Unit
Harwell, Didcot
Oxfordshire
United Kingdom

Sukarti Moeljapowiro
Laboratory of Biochemistry
Faculty of Biology
The Inter University Center for
  Biotechnology
Gadjah Mada University
Yogyakarta, Indonesia

Margaret S. Parker
Kresge Hearing Research
  Laboratory of the South

Department of
  Otorhinolaryngology and
  Biocommunication
Louisiana State University Health
  Sciences Center
New Orleans, Louisiana

Mary Z. Pelias
Department of Biometry and
  Genetics
Louisiana State University Health
  Sciences Center
New Orleans, Louisiana

Frank J. Probst
Department of Human
  Genetics
University of Michigan Medical
  School
Ann Arbor, Michigan

Yehoash Raphael
Department of Human Genetics
University of Michigan Medical
  School
Ann Arbor, Michigan

Tim J. Self
MRC Institute of Hearing
  Research
University Park, Nottingham
United Kingdom

Val C. Sheffield
The University of Iowa
Department of Pediatrics
Iowa City, Iowa

Richard J. H. Smith
The University of Iowa
Department of Otolaryngology
Iowa City, Iowa

Karen P. Steel
MRC Institute of Hearing Research
University Park, Nottingham
United Kingdom

Aihui Wang
Laboratory of Molecular Genetics
National Institute on Deafness and
  Other Communication Disorders

National Institutes of Health
Rockville, Maryland

Edward R. Wilcox
Laboratory of Molecular Genetics
National Institute on Deafness
    and Other Communication
    Disorders

National Institutes of Health
Rockville, Maryland

Sunaryana Winata
Biochemistry and Microscopic
    Anatomy
Faculty of Medicine
Udayana University
Bali, Indonesia

Of Mice and Men (and Myosins)

Karen P. Steel, Tim J. Self, Xue-Zhong Liu,
Karen B. Avraham, and Steve D. M. Brown

DEAFNESS IN HUMANS[1]

Genetic deafness is a highly heterogeneous disease: Many different genes are involved. The auditory system is highly complex, so we might expect that many different genes would be involved in its development and function. However, deafness is not a lethal condition, so mutations in many of the genes specifically involved in hearing will result in a viable individual with impaired hearing. The high degree of heterogeneity is therefore not surprising. In fact, genetic deafness is a good example of Murphy's Law: Whatever can go wrong will go wrong. The result is that deafness is the most common sensory impairment in the human population. Around 1 in 750 children have a significant, early-onset (prelingual) hearing impairment (Fortnum & Davis, 1997), and it is estimated that at least half of these impairments have a simple genetic basis. Furthermore, single gene mutations have been demonstrated to cause hearing loss with onset in adulthood in some families, and late-onset deafness with a simple genetic basis may well prove to be far more common than we presently imagine (Steel, 1998b).

Some forms of genetic deafness occur in combination with other features, allowing the disease to be defined as a specific syndrome. Over

---

[1]This chapter is based loosely on a talk presented in New Orleans in September 1998 at the Kresge Hearing Research Institute. The aim is to give a broad impression of the usefulness of the mouse as a model for studying human genetic deafness, using some examples drawn largely from our own work, rather than to present a comprehensive review of the genetics of deafness in the mouse. The chapter includes some more recently published data in addition to work presented at the talk.

400 distinct clinically defined syndromes including hearing impairment are listed in Online Mendelian Inheritance in Man (OMIM 1999; Keats & Berlin, 1999), and although hearing loss is a minor feature in some of these syndromes (e.g., Charcot-Marie-Tooth disease, osteogenesis imperfecta, etc.), in others the deafness is one of the major features. Some of the most common syndromes with deafness include Waardenburg syndrome (with pigmentary anomalies and widely spaced eyes), Treacher Collins syndrome (with craniofacial anomalies), Usher syndrome (with retinitis pigmentosa), Pendred syndrome (with goiter), Alport syndrome (with kidney defects), and branchio-oto-renal syndrome (with craniofacial and kidney defects). As these syndromes have been investigated in detail, their clinical features have sometimes led to the delineation of several discrete subtypes. Studies mapping the mutations to particular chromosomal regions led to further subdivision as it was realized that several different genes could underlie each clinical subtype. A good example of this is Usher syndrome, which was first split into type 1, with severe or profound hearing impairment, preadolescent onset of retinitis pigmentosa and balance dysfunction, and type II, which features moderate hearing impairment with later onset of retinitis pigmentosa, and no problems with balance. It was later established that a third type existed, showing progressive hearing loss, variable progression of retinitis pigmentosa and variable involvement of balance. As the responsible genes were mapped, it emerged that at least six different genes could be involved in Usher type 1, three in Usher type II, and one in Usher type III. For some of these syndromes, one or more of the responsible genes have been identified (Van Camp & Smith, 1999).

However, the majority of cases of deafness are nonsyndromic, with no obvious associated features to aid diagnosis It has for a long time been realized that there are many genes underlying nonsyndromic deafness (e.g., Morton, 1991), and early estimates of the numbers involved based on population studies suggested there were around 100. Only in the past few years have some of these been localized to particular chromosomal regions, providing evidence that many different loci are indeed involved. Over 60 loci scattered around the genome have now been defined, including dominant, recessive, X-linked, and mitochondrial modes of inheritance, and it seems likely that many further loci remain to be discovered (Van Camp & Smith, 1999). In the past 2 years there has been remarkable progress in identifying some of the genes involved, so that we now know the DNA sequence and mutations for around 15 of the genes. The types of molecules encoded by these deafness genes vary from transcription factors through channel components and motor molecules to extracellular matrix molecules (Tables 1–1 and 1–2; see Steel & Bussoli, 1999, for a review).

One surprising feature in human nonsyndromic deafness that has emerged in the past couple of years is the preponderance of mutations in the *GJB2* gene, encoding connexin 26, in some populations. Western pop-

Table 1–1. Some molecules involved in nonsyndromic deafness.

Molecule	Inheritance	Type of Protein
Connexin 26	Dom+Rec	Channel component
Connexin 31	Dom+Rec	Channel component
Connexin 30	Dom	Channel component
KCNQ4	Dom	Channel component
Pendrin	Rec+Pendred	Ion transporter
Myosin 7A	Dom+Rec+Usher	Motor molecule
Myosin 15	Rec	Motor molecule
Diaphanous	Dom	Cytoskeletal protein
POU3F4	X-linked Rec	Transcription factor
POU4F3	Dom	Transcription factor
α-tectorin	Dom+Rec	Extracellular matrix
Coch	Dom	Extracellular matrix
Otoferlin	Rec	Synapse component
DFNA5	Dom	Novel

Note: See Steel and Bussoli (1999) for references and further details. Dom = dominant, Rec = recessive.

Table 1–2. Some molecules involved in syndromic deafness.

Molecule	Other Affected Sites	Syndrome	Type of Protein
Connexin 32	Peripheral nerves	CMT	Channel component
ATP6B1	Kidney	RTA	Ion pump
Pendrin	Thyroid	Pendred	Ion transporter
KVLQT1	Heart	JLS	Channel component
KCNE1	Heart	JLS	Channel component
Myosin 7A	Retina	Usher 1B	Motor molecule
EYA1	Kidney, jaw	BOR	Transcription factor
PAX3	Pigmentation	WS1	Transcription factor
MITF	Pigmentation	WS2	Transcription factor
SOX10	Pigmentation, gut	WS4	Transcription factor
EDNRB	Pigmentation, gut	WS4	Receptor
EDN3	Pigmentation, gut	WS4	Ligand
FGFR3	Skull	CSS	Receptor
Treacle	Skull and jaw	TCS	Trafficking protein
Norrin	Eye, brain	Norrie	Extracellular matrix
USH2A	Retina	Usher 2A	Extracellular matrix
Collagens 4	Kidney	Alport	Extracellular matrix
Collagen 2	Eye, joints, palate	Stickler	Extracellular matrix
DDP	Muscle	DFN1	Mitochondrial protein

Note: See Steel and Bussoli (1999) for references and further details.

ulations seem to have relatively high frequencies of *GJB2* mutations, especially the 35delG mutation. In Spanish and Italian populations this gene may account for up to 50% of cases of recessive nonsyndromic childhood deafness (e.g., Denoyelle et al., 1997; Estivill et al., 1998; Kelley et al., 1998; Morell et al., 1998; Zelante et al., 1997). In contrast, this gene is rarely involved in deafness in Asian populations. The small size of the gene, which makes screening for mutations relatively simple, together with the relatively high frequency of mutations in some populations makes molecular testing a viable option to aid diagnosis and genetic counselling when this is sought. However, there are a number of uncertainties in interpreting the results of mutation screening, making it necessary to act with considerable caution in predicting the hearing status of newborn or unborn children on the basis of molecular tests, at least until we understand more about the reasons for the variability (e.g., Steel 1998a; Denoyelle et al., 1999).

WHY MICE?

Despite the progress in identifying deafness genes in humans outlined above, it is very difficult to establish the mechanisms directly involved in hearing impairment in humans. If we are ever to devise treatments for hearing impairment, it will be necessary to understand the biological basis of the disorder, and mice are ideal models for moving toward this goal. Many approaches that are not feasible in humans can be used in mice, such as making a detailed study of the development of the defect to establish the site of the earliest anomalies, performing invasive electrophysiological investigations like measuring endocochlear potentials or single hair cell studies, using a genetic approach to define a region containing a deafness gene by making a congenic region by targeted breeding, or carrying out experimental manipulations such as knocking out a particular gene or introducing a specific mutation into the genome. These techniques can be used to dissect the pathological process and are so useful that, whenever a deafness gene is identified in humans and there appears to be no homologous mouse mutant, transgenic techniques are used to create a suitable model mouse. Furthermore, mice have proven very helpful in providing candidate genes for involvement in human deafness, and several human deafness genes have been identified only after the gene was identified in a deaf mouse mutant (e.g., Waardenburg syndrome types I and II, Usher syndrome 1B, DFNB3, DFNA15; see Probst & Camper, 1999, for references).

Mice are thus very useful for studying the biological basis of genetic deafness, but are they good models for human deafness? The answer is with very few exceptions yes. The mammalian inner ear is unlike that of any other vertebrate in having a highly specialized cochlea with inner and outer hair cells, specialized supporting cells reinforced with microtubule bundles, and a pigmented stria vascularis that generates a high resting potential, the endocochlear potential, in the fluid bathing the sensory hair cells. Therefore, a model system should ideally be a mammal, and the mouse is the obvious choice, having a cochlea that is virtually identical (except in size) to that of humans. The mouse and human genomes are both well-characterized, and the similarities are extensive, suggesting that genes identified in the mouse will almost always have a human orthologue, and vice versa. Many mouse mutants with defects of the auditory system are already in existence, and many of these have associated features making them comparable to human deafness syndromes. Thus, there are both humans and mice with deafness with pigmentary anomalies, with skeletal malformations like digit defects, with pinna malformations, or with other craniofacial anomalies. Deaf mouse mutants are also similar to humans in the broad range of types of auditory defect observed, insofar as this can be determined in humans. For example, both mice and humans can have primary conductive defects due to middle ear malformations, gross malformations of the whole or part of the labyrinth, primary organ of Corti defects, primary dysfunction of endolymph production, or hearing impairment due to a central auditory system abnormality. These observations suggest that the same biological processes are highly likely to be involved in the two species, making the mouse a good model. In the few cases where mice and humans with mutations in the equivalent deafness gene differ in their phenotype, the reasons for these differences can be trivial and unrelated to hearing impairment (e.g., the homozygous *Gjb2* mutant mouse dies early in development because of differences in placental structure compared with humans, while GJB2 mutations are a common cause of recessive deafness in humans), or the differences can be potentially instructive in pointing to factors such as modifier genes that alter the expression of a mutant gene but are present as different alleles in the two species (e.g., Steel & Smith, 1992).

Despite the value of deaf mouse mutants for understanding human hereditary deafness, the full potential of using them as models has not yet been realized. Indeed, if we line up comparable stretches of mouse and human chromosomes, there is often no deaf mouse mutant corresponding to a particular human deafness locus, suggesting that we have not yet found the mouse model for that form of human deafness. This is a problem that we will return to at the end of the chapter. Likewise, among the deafness genes identified in the mouse, not all have an obvious human homologue, which is perhaps not surprising because to date the mutations responsible for only a small proportion of the cases of human genetic deafness have been localized or identified.

In this chapter, we will take just a few selected examples of how deaf mutant mice have been used to advance our understanding of the pathological processes in the ear in genetic deafness, as an illustration of the sorts of approaches that might be useful in our long-term goal of developing treatment strategies for human hereditary deafness. Several recent reviews cover a broader range of mouse models for hereditary deafness (Bussoli & Steel, 1999; Fekete 1999; Holme & Steel, 1999; Kiernan & Steel, 2000; Probst & Camper, 1999; Steel, 1995.)

MYOSINS AND DEAFNESS

Shaker1

Two of the earliest deafness genes to be identified as affecting sensory hair cells turned out to encode unconventional myosin molecules, and both were found by positional cloning of mutations in deaf mouse mutants. The first of these was the *Myo7a* gene, encoding myosin VIIA (Gibson et al., 1995). *Myo7a* was found to be mutated in several alleles of the *shaker 1* mutant, a classic deaf mouse mutant first described in the 1920s by Lord and Gates (1929). *Shaker 1* mice show deafness and balance defects leading to hyperactivity, head-tossing, and circling behavior, and had previously been reported to show progressive degeneration of both cochlear and vestibular hair cells (Deol, 1956). Several other mutations at the same locus have been discovered over the past few years, and although a number of these have been lost, at least nine are available in addition to the original mutation. The overt balance defects make new mutations easy to detect, which along with the relatively large size of the gene probably accounts for the large number of alleles.

Myosin VIIA is a very large molecule of 2,215 amino acids. Mutations have been determined in seven sh1 alleles in total, including the original spontaneous mutation, one further spontaneous mutation, and five ENU-induced mutations (Gibson et al., 1995; Mburu et al., 1997; see Table 1–3). ENU (*N*-ethyl-*N*-nitrosourea) is a powerful mutagen that leads to single base changes, and the two spontaneous mutations also are single base changes. Five of the mutations occur in the 5′ part of the gene coding for the motor domain of the molecule, a region that is conserved among all myosins and contains the actin-binding and ATP-binding regions, and two mutations affect the tail domain, the most divergent part of the myosin molecule, thought to determine the specificity of the myosin for interactions with other molecules (Figure 1–1). The amounts of myosin VIIA in kidney and testis, two organs that express the *Myo7a* gene, vary between alleles from near-normal levels in the original allele to effective nulls in two of the mutations (Hasson, Walsh, et al., 1997; Liu, Udovichenko, Brown, Steel, & Williams, 1999; Table 1–3), and we assume that similar levels are present in the inner ears of these mutants. The reduced amounts of myosin VIIA produced from the mutant alleles may contribute to their effects on phenotype, in addition to the effects of the mutation on any myosin produced. However, heterozygotes for all seven alleles studied show normal hearing, suggesting that 50% of the normal amount of myosin VIIA is sufficient for hair cells to function.

Table 1–3. *Shaker 1* mutations and resulting protein levels.

Allele	Mutation	Protein Level
*Myo7a*sh1	CGG→CCG Arg502Pro	93%
*Myo7a*6J	CGT→CCT Arg241Pro	21%
*Myo7a*26SB	TTT→ATT Phe1800Ile	18–46%
*Myo7a*3336SB	TGT→TGA Cys2182stop	13%
*Myo7a*816SB	IVS16nt-2a→g del (646-655)	6.3%
*Myo7a*4494SB	IVS6nt+2t→a→ stop 5aa downstream	<1%
*Myo7a*4626SB	CAG→TAG Gln720stop	<1%

Note: Mutations are from Mburu et al. (1997) and protein levels are from kidney and testis (Hasson, Walsh, et al., 1997b).

Myosin VIIA is found in several tissues, including kidney, testis, lung, retina and hair cells of the inner ear (El-Amraoui et al., 1996; Gibson et al., 1995; Hasson, Heintzelman, Santos-Sacchi, Corey, & Mooseker, 1995; Hasson, Gillespie, et al., 1997; Hasson, Walsh, et al., 1997; Liu, Vansant, et al., 1997), but there are no obvious kidney, testis, or lung abnormalities in humans or mice with *Myo7a* mutations. In the retina, myosin VIIA is located in the pigmented retinal epithelium and the connecting cilium of photoreceptor cells (El-Amraoui et al., 1996; Liu, Ondek, & Williams, 1998; Liu, Vasant, et al., 1997). In hair cells of the inner ear, myosin VIIA is located in the cytoplasm and cuticular plate, and was found to be particularly concentrated within the vesicle-rich region around the cuticular plate (the pericuticular necklace), and at the membranes of the stereocilia (Hasson, Gillespie, et al., 1997).

Myosin VIIA Mutations in Humans

The human version of the myosin VIIA gene, MYO7A, was found to be mutated in humans with Usher syndrome type 1B shortly after the identification of the mouse gene (Weil et al., 1995). Usher syndrome 1B involves severe or profound congenital hearing impairment, balance dysfunction, and progressive retinitis pigmentosa starting before adolescence. This phenotype corresponds to the hearing and balance defects in *shaker 1* mice, but the mouse mutants do not show any obvious retinal degeneration during

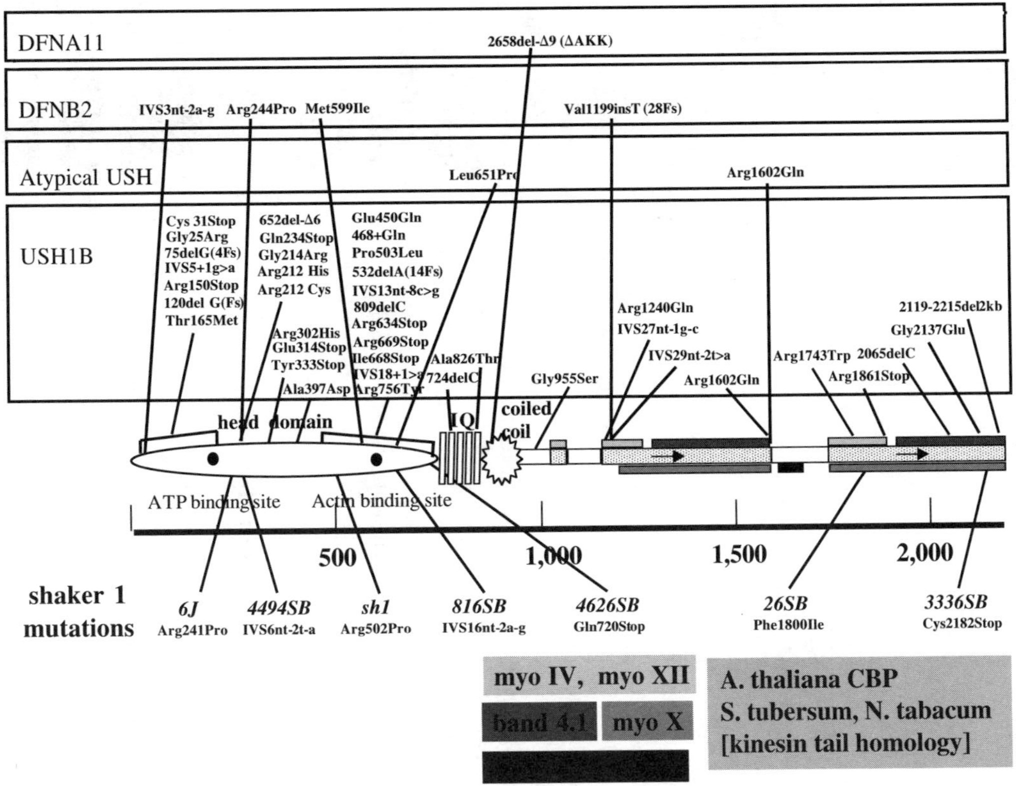

Figure 1–1. Spectrum of *MYO7A* mutations that lead to Usher syndrome type 1B, atypical Usher syndrome, nonsyndromic dominant and recessive deafness (see Liu, Hope, et al., 1998, for details of sources). The horizontal bar in the middle represents the myosin VIIA molecule, with the motor head domain on the left (dark spots indicating the ATP binding site and the actin binding site), followed by the IQ domain and the coiled coil region, and the tail domain on the right, with different shaded bars indicating regions of sequence similarity (key to shade coding is given at the bottom). The position of the seven known shaker1 mouse mutations are shown at the bottom, and the human mutations at the top. Scale bar represents numbers of amino acids. (Reprinted with permission from "Mutations in the Myosin VIIA Gene Cause a Wide Phenotypie Spectrum Including Atypical Usher Syndrome," by Liu, Hope, et al., 1998, Fig. 2, *American Journal of Human Genetics, 63,* 909–912. Copyright 1998 University of Chicago Press.)

their 2-year lifespan (Hasson, Walsh, et al., 1997). This may be due to the fact that mice do not live long enough to develop retinal degeneration. Recent work suggests that there may be anomalous opsin transport through the connecting cilium of photoreceptor cells in *Myo7a* mutant mice, and if this was also the case in humans, one could imagine that it could lead to increased vulnerability of the photoreceptors to damage in the longer term (Liu et al., 1999).

However, since the original finding of MYO7A mutations in Usher syndrome 1B, mutations in the same gene have been found in three other types of human hearing impairment: atypical Usher syndrome, with variable and progressive hearing impairment, variable involvement of the vestibular system, and later onset of retinitis pigmentosa than in Usher 1B; nonsyndromic recessive deafness (DFNB2), with no sign of visual defects; and nonsyndromic dominant deafness (DFNA11), again with no evidence of involvement of the retina (Liu, Hope, et al., 1998; Liu, Walsh, Mburu, et al., 1997, Liu, Walsh, Tamagawa, et al., 1997; Weil et al., 1997). There is no particular pattern of genotype/phenotype correlation, and mutations in cases of nonsyndromic deafness are interspersed with Usher 1B mutations along the whole length of the gene (Figure 1–1). An exception to this is the one dominantly inherited mutation, a 9-bp deletion found in the family defining the DFNA11 locus, which is the only mutation so far detected in the coiled coil domain of the gene (Liu, Walsh, Tomagawa, et al., 1997). Myosin VIIA has been shown to self-associate (Weil et al., 1997), presumably by dimerizing at the coiled coil region, and interference with the dimerization process may endow the mutant protein with a dominant effect.

The finding of nonsyndromic as well as syndromic forms of deafness in people with MYO7A mutations suggests another possible explanation for the lack of overt retinal degeneration in *shaker 1* mutants: The effects of MYO7A mutations on the retina may be moderated by interactions with other genes elsewhere in the genome. These modifier genes are presumed to have different alleles, some of which ameliorate the deleterious effects of the mutation on the retina (as in human nonsyndromic deafness and shaker1 mutants), while others cannot rescue the retinal effects (as in Usher syndrome). The importance of this phenomenon, if it turns out to be the mechanism explaining the variation among humans and mice with MYO7A mutations, is that identifying the modifiers could provide clues to the ultimate prevention of the retinal effects. For example, an advantageous modifier gene could be upregulated, or a disadvantageous modifier could be downregulated, or knowledge of the molecular basis of the retinal degeneration could lead to the development of other forms of drug-based treatment. Furthermore, the same modifiers might determine whether the hearing impairment is congenital and stable, or is progressive, and similar interventions could be envisaged to stop the progression of the latter type. There is some evidence from the mouse to suggest that modifiers may influence the effects of the original, mildest *Myo7a* mutation so far characterized (*Myo7a^{sh1}*), in that changing the genetic background of this mutation alters the progression of the hearing loss and leads to histological differences in the organ of Corti (Deol, 1956; Emmerling & Sobkowicz, 1990).

Role of Myosin VIIA in Hair Cell Development and Function

What are the effects of *Myo7a* mutations upon the development of cochlear hair cells in the shaker1 mouse mutants? We have investigated this using scanning and transmission electron microscopy in three of the alleles, *Myo7a^{sh1}*, *Myo7a^{6J}*, and *Myo7a^{816SB}* (see Table 1–3; Self et al., 1998). The effects are most clearly seen by scanning electron microscopy of the surface of the hair cells (Figure 1–2). In the mildest of the mutations, *Myo7a^{sh1}*, which has a missense arginine to proline mutation affecting an unconserved surface loop of the molecule (Table 1–3), the stereocilia bundles develop apparently normally, but by around 15 days after birth, only two rows of stereocilia can be seen instead of the more usual three rows in outer hair cells (Figure 1–2A and B). From this time onwards, hair cells progressively degenerate (Self et al., 1998). In a more severe allele, *Myo7a^{6J}*, which has a missense arginine to proline mutation affecting a key amino acid residue at the core of the motor domain (Table 1–3), the stereocilia bundles become disorganized. As the hair cells can first be distinguished from their surrounding supporting cells at around 16.5 to 17.5 days of gestation, they appear to be normally polarized, with the kinocilium always located at the lateral edge of the cell. By 18.5 days, the developing stereocilia also appear to be generally polarized correctly, with the longest stereocilia starting to grow in a crescent arrangement at the lateral pole of the cell, but early signs of disorganization can be detected in the homozygous mutants. By 3 days after birth, the stereocilia in controls form a neat V-shaped array, but in the mutants they are grossly disorganized within the top of the hair cell, with small clusters arranged in abnormal orientations (Figure 1–2C and D). These mutant stereocilia do show some normal features, in having grown to form rows of graded heights, and tip links and cross links can be observed between adjacent stereocilia, but their position in the top of the hair cell is clearly abnormal. By 20 days after birth, these hair cells are losing their stereocilia and starting to disappear. A third mutant allele was studied, *Myo7a^{816SB}*, which has a splice-site mutation leading to exon-skipping and predicted deletion of 10 amino acids in the motor domain (Table 1–3). In this allele, the disorganization of the stereocilia bundles appeared to be even more severe than in the *Myo7a^{6J}* mutation (Figure 1–2E and F).

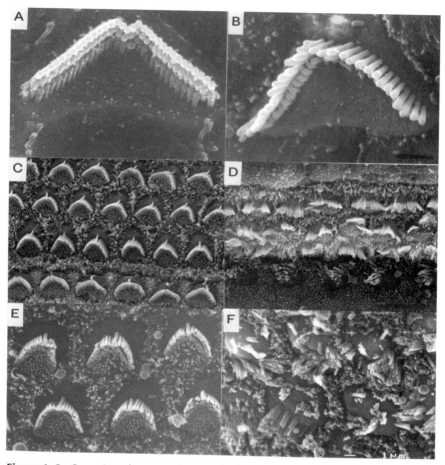

Figure 1–2. Scanning electron micrographs from three different *shaker 1* alleles. **A.** Control outer hair cell stereocilia bundle at 15 days after birth, showing three rows of stereocilia. **B.** *Myo7a^{sh1}/Myo7a^{sh1}* mutant outer hair cell bundle, showing only two rows of stereocilia. **C.** Control organ of Corti at 3 days old. **D.** Littermate *Myo7a^{6J}/Myo7a^{6J}* mutant at 3 days old, showing disorganized hair bundles. **E.** Two rows of outer hair cells from a control mouse at 3 days after birth. **F.** Two rows of outer hair cells from a mutant *Myo7a^{816SB}/Myo7a^{816SB}* cochlea, with extensive disorganization of the stereocilia bundles.

Scale bars represent: A,B 1μm, C,D 10μm, E,F 1μm.

Can the pathology of the *shaker 1* mutants tell us anything about the role of myosin VIIA in hair cells? We have addressed several possible functions by examining the mutants. First, we wondered if myosin VIIA might be involved in the condensation of the cuticular plate, which appears

shortly before birth as a dense, organelle-free plate below the apical surface of the hair cells, anchoring the rootlets of the stereocilia. If there is a
delay or abnormality in the condensation of this plate, then the stereocilia
might be free to move around within the top of the hair cell rather than become anchored to form the V-shaped array. Transmission electron microscopy of developing hair cells in the mutants showed that the cuticular
plate did condense at the correct time, suggesting this hypothesis was not
the explanation for the disorganization of stereocilia bundles (Self et al.,
1998). Furthermore, there was no obvious difference in the ultrastructural
relationship between stereocilia rootlets and the dense material of the cuticular plate, so there was no indication from this approach that the stereocilia were more loosely anchored in the cuticular plate than normal.

Second, the apical surface of hair cells appears to be a region of much
endocytotic and exocytotic activity, and the resulting membrane turnover
could control the position of the stereocilia, so we investigated whether
there was evidence for a difference in this activity between mutants and
controls that might account for the disorganization. Transmission electron
microscopy showed the presence of endocytotic pits at the apical surfaces
of both mutant and control hair cells, and freeze-fracture of apical profiles
also showed ample pits in mutants (Richardson et al., 1997). When these
freeze-fracture images were quantified, there was no difference in the
numbers of pits on each hair cell between mutants and controls, arguing
against this hypothesis (Table 1–4). However, the total apical surface area
of mutant hair cells was significantly greater than in controls, which could
indicate that membrane turnover was not completely normal in mutants
(Table 1–4; Richardson et al., 1997). A further indication that membrane
processes were not quite normal in mutants came from the observation
that radiolabeled aminoglycoside antibiotics were not taken up in large
quantities by mutant hair cells, whereas normal hair cells seem specifically
to take up these drugs (Richardson et al., 1997). The explanation for the
lack of uptake of aminoglycosides by $Myo7a^{6J}$ mutant hair cells is not obvious (see Richardson et al., 1997, for discussion), but the finding clearly im-
plicates myosin VIIA in the process. Finally, ferritin uptake by $Myo7a^{6J}$ mutant hair cells in organ culture was normal, indicating that fluid-phase

Table 1–4. Endocytotic pits in apical profiles of basal OHCs in culture.

	Pits per Apex	Apex Area, μ^2	Pits per μ^2
+/$Myo7a^{6J}$	102±42	38±10	2.73±0.84
$Myo7a^{6J}$/$Myo7a^{6J}$	97±25	46±9*	2.17±0.58*

*Significantly different from heterozygote ($p<0.05$); n = 29 and 25.
Source: Data from Richardson et al. (1997).

uptake was probably normal, in contrast to the aminoglycoside uptake, which was not normal (Richardson et al., 1997). This difference could result from different mechanisms of uptake, with ferritin being taken up in a nonspecific manner and aminoglycosides being taken up by specific receptors which in turn depend on normal myosin VIIA function (Richardson et al., 1997). In summary, there is little evidence for a general abnormality in membrane turnover at the apical surface of $Myo7a^{6J}$ hair cells that could account for the stereocilia disorganization.

Third, we examined carefully the relationship between the kinocilium and the arrangement of the stereocilia bundle, because the location of the kinocilium at the point of the V-shape led previous investigators to speculate that the kinocilium might control bundle formation. As already mentioned, the kinocilium appears to be correctly located at the lateral pole of the hair cells from the earliest stages studied. However, in the $Myo7a^{6J}$ and $Myo7a^{816SB}$ mutants at 3 days after birth, we saw no obvious relationship between the position of the kinocilium and the clusters of stereocilia, indicating that either the kinocilium has no role in organizing the stereocilia bundle or that it requires functional myosin VIIA molecules to carry out this role.

Fourth, we investigated the suggestion that myosin VIIA might provide the intracellular anchor of cross links between adjacent stereocilia (Hasson, Gillespie, et al., 1997). The reason for this hypothesis was that myosin VIIA was found to be enriched at the membranes of stereocilia, and in frog sacculus hair cells it was particularly concentrated in a band just above the basal tapers, corresponding to the location of a particular type of interstereocilia link called the ankle link (Hasson, Gillespie, et al., 1997a). In mammals, these ankle links are distributed along the length of the stereocilium rather than being concentrated near the ankles, and myosin VIIA is also evenly distributed along the stereocilium. If these crosslinks between adjacent stereocilia were abnormal in some way in the shaker1 mutants, this could possibly lead to drifting apart of clusters of stereocilia as we observed in some of the shaker1 alleles. We looked at crosslinks qualitatively by field emission electron microscopy, and found no obvious differences between $Myo7a^{6J}$or $Myo7a^{sh1}$ mutants and controls in the appearance of these links. We also examined ultrathin sections across the stereocilia bundle and measured distances between stereocilia within clusters in $Myo7a^{6J}$ mutants and compared these with controls, but there was no significant difference in spacing between mutants and controls (Self & Steel, unpublished data). These observations did not support the suggestion that crosslinks might be the mediator of stereocilia bundle disorganization, at least in the $Myo7a^{6J}$ allele.

Thus, we have not yet been able to establish decisively the role of myosin VIIA in hair cell development, but we have succeeded in ruling out some of the more obvious hypotheses to explain the disorganized hair bundle. What of hair cell function? Gross recordings of compound action potentials, cochlear microphonics, and summating potentials in the three alleles described above correlated broadly with the ultrastructural observations. The two most severely affected alleles, $Myo7a^{6J}$ and $Myo7a^{816SB}$, showed very little or no response to tone-burst stimuli, while the original sh1 allele, $Myo7a^{sh1}$, which has the mildest ultrastructural defects of the alleles studied, showed some responses for a short period after the normal time of onset around 12 to 14 days after birth, although these were never of normal threshold and quickly deteriorated as the mutants aged (Harvey 1989; Self et al., 1998; Steel & Harvey, 1992). However, measurements of transducer currents from single outer hair cells in organ culture at 1 to 3 days after birth revealed that, at this stage, transducer currents could be obtained from $Myo7a^{6J}$ mutants and were of similar size to those obtained from controls (Richardson et al., 1997). Single hair cell recordings from neonatal cultured specimens are likely to be very helpful in understanding the role not only of myosin VIIA but also of other molecules involved in genetic deafness where hair cells seem to be the primary target of the mutations.

Snell's Waltzer

The second gene to be identified as affecting hair cells directly surprisingly also turned out to encode an unconventional myosin molecule, myosin VI. The mutant is *Snell's waltzer*, another of the classic deaf mouse mutants, first described by Deol and Green in 1966. It shows progressive hair cell loss and deafness, combined with hyperactivity, head-tossing, and circling indicative of vestibular dysfunction. The myosin VI gene, *Myo6*, was identified by positional cloning, and an intragenic deletion of 130 bp was discovered in the mutant allele, leading to a frameshift and predicted truncation of the product (Avraham et al., 1995). No myosin VI protein could be detected in any tissue, suggesting it is a null allele. A second allele involved an inversion associated with greatly reduced myosin VI protein levels, but this allele has not been so well characterized so we describe only the original allele below. The human MYO6 gene has been isolated, but no mutations in families with hearing impairment have yet been discovered (Avraham et al., 1997).

Myosin VI is widely expressed in many tissues, but only inner ear defects have been noted in *Snell's waltzer* mutants, suggesting that the myosin VI molecule is redundant in other locations (Avraham et al., 1995; Buss et al., 1998; Hasson, Gillespie et al., 1997). In the inner ear, myosin VI is found in hair cells and is particularly concentrated in the vesicle-rich pericuticular necklace and in the cuticular plate (Hasson, Gillespie et al.,

1997). In mammals, it was not detected in stereocilia, and the recent report that myosin VI runs in the opposite direction along actin filaments (toward the minus end) compared with other myosin molecules might explain why it does not enter stereocilia while other hair cell myosins do (Wells et al., 1999).

We have looked at the *Snell's waltzer* cochlea to investigate the role of myosin VI in hair cell development (Self et al., 1999). Like myosin VIIA, myosin VI is involved in the development of stereocilia bundles, but the mechanism seems to be different, with early stereocilia fusion being a prominent feature. In *Snell's waltzer* hair cells at birth, stereocilia bundles appear largely normal, with the tallest stereocilia arranged in a crescent shape at the lateral edge of the cell apex, but minor signs of disorganization (a "swirling" appearance) can be found in a few cells. Transmission electron microscopy at this stage shows a few places where apical hair cell membranes are slightly raised between adjacent stereocilia (Self et al., 1999). One day later, more of the hair bundles are disorganized, and signs of fusion can be seen by scanning electron microscopy. By 3 days after birth, extensive fusion can be seen, associated with obvious disorganization of bundles (Figure 1–3A and B). The fusion appears to start at the base and progress toward the tips of the stereocilia, as if the membranes are zipping up. By 7 days, most hair cells have only a few fused stereocilia (Figure 1–3 C–F), and these continue to fuse and also grow in length, so that by 20 days the hair cells sport giant fused stereocilia, sometimes with swellings at or near their tips (Figure 1–4) (Self et al., 1999).

The fusion of membranes between stereocilia seems to be the major pathological feature in *Snell's waltzer*, and could presumably account for the other observed changes (disorganization and swirling of bundles, growth of giant stereocilia, ultimate degeneration of hair cells). We have considered several possible explanations for the fusion. First, abnormal membrane turnover might lead to a net loss of apical membrane, and consequent pulling up of membrane between stereocilia. This seems unlikely, because stereocilia continue to grow during the period studied, rather than being forced back into the cell to minimize apical membrane area. Furthermore, we see no evidence of abnormal membrane turnover in mutant hair cells: Endocytotic pits of normal ultrastructural appearance are detected at the apical surface, and the membrane dye FM1-43 is taken up by mutant as well as by control hair cells, suggesting active endocytosis occurs in mutants, although neither of these approaches was quantified (Self et al., 1999).

A second explanation might be that myosin VI could serve to anchor the stereocilia rootlets into the cuticular plate, and in its absence the stereocilia could pull out of the plate, dragging membrane with them. This also

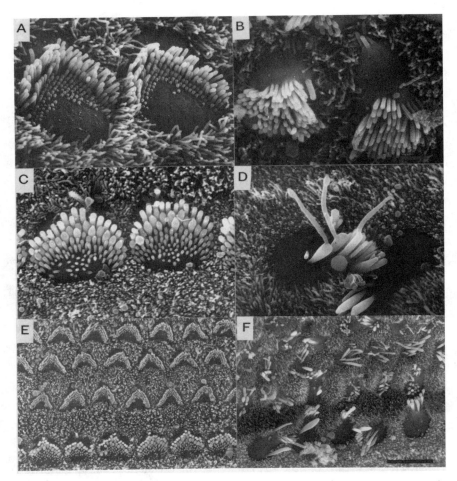

Figure 1–3. Scanning electron micrographs of the *Snell's waltzer* mouse mutant. **A.** Control outer hair cells at 3 days of age. **B.** *Myo6^{sv}/Myo6^{sv}* mutant outer hair cells, showing fusion of stereocilia starting from the base, and disorganization of the bundle. **C.** Control inner hair cells from a 7-day-old mouse. **D.** *Myo6^{sv}/Myo6^{sv}* mutant inner hair cells, showing further fusion of stereocilia and excess growth. **E.** Control organ of Corti at 7 days old. **F.** *Myo6^{sv}/Myo6^{sv}* organ of Corti at 7 days of age, showing extensive disorganization and fusion of stereocilia bundles in all rows of hair cells.

Scale bars represent: A,B,C,D, 1μm, E,F, 10μm.

seems an unlikely explanation, because we might expect the stereocilia to appear to extend (by scanning electron microscopy of the upper surface of the hair cell) before the fusion is observed, but instead we see fusion prior

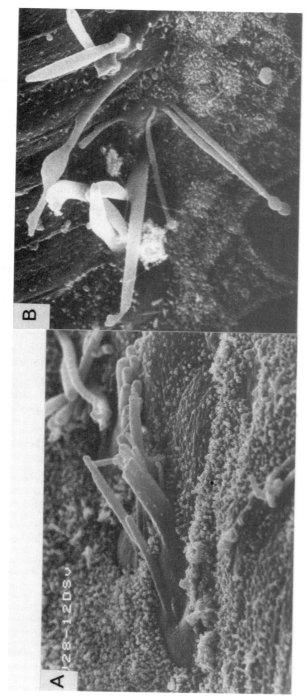

Figure 1–4. Scanning electron micrographs of further *Snell's waltzer* hair cells. **A.** 12-day-old mutant inner hair cells. **B.** 20-day-old mutant inner hair cells, showing the growth of giant stereocilia.

Scale bar represents 1 μm.

to extension. Furthermore, we saw no obvious detachment of stereocilia rootlets by transmission electron microscopy in neonatal stages.

Third, myosin VI might be involved in the delivery of components to the growing stereocilia, because unconventional myosins are often assumed to have a primary cargo-carrying role, and in the *Drosophila* embryo, the myosin VI homologue has been shown directly to mediate vesicle transport (Mermall, McNally, & Miller, 1994; Mermall, Post, & Mooseker, 1998). If the delivery of stereocilia components is not properly balanced, the result might be the uncontrolled growth of stereocilia that we observe. However, it is difficult to imagine how this explanation could account for the initial fusion of membranes.

Our fourth and favored hypothesis is that myosin VI might normally be involved in anchoring the apical cell membrane to the actin in the cuticular plate (Self et al., 1999). In this model, the motor end of the myosin VI molecule would attach to the abundant actin in the cuticular plate, while the tail of the myosin would attach directly or indirectly to the apical membrane, serving to hold down the membrane between adjacent stereocilia. The natural tendency of a lipid-rich cell membrane in an aqueous environment would be to form a sphere with a minimal surface area to minimize surface tension, and any other configuration must be actively maintained. The arrangement of stereocilia, with closely apposed membranes, seems likely to require very active maintenance to avoid the tendency to fusion. In the absence of adequate anchoring, the membranes between stereocilia may proceed to zip up, rising to the tops of the stereocilia and leading to fusion. This explanation does not account for the continued growth of stereocilia to form giant protrusions on the apical surface, but once fusion has started, the whole process of stereocilia growth and maintenance will likely be disrupted, and the excess growth may be secondary to the fusion.

In summary, the myosin VI molecule appears to have a role in hair cell development and function that is distinct from the role of myosin VIIA, as might be expected from the fact that both are essential molecules for normal cochlear function. A further unconventional myosin, myosin XV (*Myo15*), has more recently also been discovered to underlie both mouse and human deafness, in the *shaker 2* mouse mutant and the recessive deafness DFNB3 (Probst et al., 1998; Wang et al., 1998). In the *shaker 2* mutants, a further distinct stereocilia defect is found: They are much shorter than normal. These three molecules are among the first that have been demonstrated to have an essential role in hair cells and represent the start of the process of unraveling the molecular basis of auditory function. In contrast to the visual or olfactory systems, we know very little about the molecular basis of hair cell function, and a genetic approach is proving to be very helpful in identifying essential molecular components.

IONIC HOMEOSTASIS IN
THE COCHLEAR DUCT

It is perhaps not surprising that there has been a great deal of focus on hair cells, and in particular hair cell degeneration, in investigating the cellular basis of hearing impairment. Much effort in the past has been expended in counting degenerating and missing hair cells and correlating these counts with auditory function. With the extended use of more detailed ways of assessing the state of the cochlear duct, such as scanning and transmission electron microscopy, it has become clear that hair cell degeneration is rarely, if ever, the cause of hearing impairment in hereditary deafness, but that instead the hair cells may have distinct developmental or functional defects that cause the hearing impairment and lead to secondary hair cell degeneration.

However, one of the striking realizations from the research in both human and mouse genetic deafness over the past few years has been the importance of the rest of the cochlear duct, and in particular the roles of different cell types in maintaining cochlear homeostasis (Steel & Bussoli, 1999). It is not a new observation that the stria vascularis is important for cochlear function (e.g., Schuknecht, 1974; Steel & Bock, 1983), but the number of different deafness genes that appear to have a primary role in homeostasis is surprisingly larger than the number so far identified that affect hair cells directly (Steel & Bussoli, 1999). This is an area where work on animal models has been critical to understanding the processes involved, because, for example, measuring the resting potential (the endocochlear potential, normally around 80 to 100 mV) in the endolymph bathing the upper surfaces of the sensory hair cells is too invasive to be carried out in humans, yet it provides key information about the functional basis of the deafness.

Endocochlear potential is necessary for normal hair cell function in the mammalian cochlea, as it provides a large potential difference across the top of the hair cells, from the positive potential in scala media to the negative interior of the hair cell, and animals with reduced or absent endocochlear potentials have raised thresholds for cochlear responses. The potential is generated by the stria vascularis on the lateral wall of the cochlear duct and depends also on adequate electrical resistance of the boundaries of scala media. It is an electrogenic potential generated by the pumping of potassium ions into scala media by the stria. Endolymph has a high potassium, low sodium content, and it is thought that, when the transducer channels in the sensory hair cells are opened by sound stimulation, the current passing into the cell down the electrical gradient is mostly carried by potassium, as it is the predominant cation available. It is believed that the potassium flowing into the hair cells is recycled through the supporting cells and fibrocytes of the cochlear duct, back to the stria vascularis for pumping back into the endolymph (e.g., Kikuchi, Kimura, Paul, & Adams, 1995; Spicer & Schulte, 1996) (Figure 1–5). The ionic composition of the endolymph and the endocochlear potential are to some extent separate aspects of the system, as the high potassium content is established before the endocochlear potential during development, and vestibular endolymph has a similar high potassium, low sodium content but has no high resting potential like cochlear endolymph.

The first attempts to record endocochlear potentials in animal models of hereditary deafness with strial defects were reported by Suga and Hattler, who looked at two deaf white cats and three deaf dalmatian dogs, and failed to record any endocochlear potential (Suga & Hattler 1970). However, the Reissner's membrane had collapsed extensively in these animals, and there was no indication that the recording electrode had actually passed through the small remaining open area of scala media. Later measurements of a reduced or absent endocochlear potential in the viable dominant spotting mouse mutant (W^v/W^v, since identified as the *Kit* gene encoding a growth factor) were corroborated by serial 1 micron-thick sections through the cochlea, to show that the hole in the lateral wall of the cochlear duct made by the recording electrode did open into an open scala media (Steel & Barkway, 1989; Steel, Barkway, & Bock, 1987). Since these early reports, several other mouse mutants have been shown to have an open scala media but a reduced or absent endocochlear potential, such as further alleles of the *Kit* gene (Cable, Huszar, Jaenisch, & Steel, 1994), the steel-dickie mutant (Sl^d, since identified as the ligand of the *Kit* growth factor, *Mgf*; Steel, Davidson, & Jackson, 1992), the light allele of brown (*Tyrp1^{lt}*; Cable, Jackson, & Steel, 1993), the varitint-waddler mutant (*Va^J*; Cable & Steel, 1998), and most recently the *Pou3f4* mouse mutant (Minowa et al., 1999; Steel, 1999).

The *Kit*, *Mgf*, *Va^J*, and *Tyrp1^{lt}* mouse mutants mentioned above have in common pigmentation anomalies, such that parts or all of their bodies are devoid of the pigment cells, melanocytes, leading to white coats and also to a lack of melanocytes in the stria vascularis in their cochleas. The cells themselves are missing, rather than being present but unable to produce pigment as in albinos, and we have demonstrated in the *Kit* and *Mgf* mutant alleles we studied that the precursors of these melanocytes migrate from the neural crest as usual, but then frequently fail to survive when they reach their target tissue, such as the inner ear (Cable, Jackson, & Steel, 1995; Steel et al., 1992). The absence of melanocytes is invariably associated with absence of endocochlear potential, suggesting a causative relationship (Cable, Huszar, Jaenisch, & Steel, 1994). Melanocyte-like cells form the intermediate cells of the stria, scattered between the marginal cells on the lumenal side and the basal cells adjacent to the fibrocytes forming the outer wall of the cochlear duct. Their role in generating the endocochlear potential is not

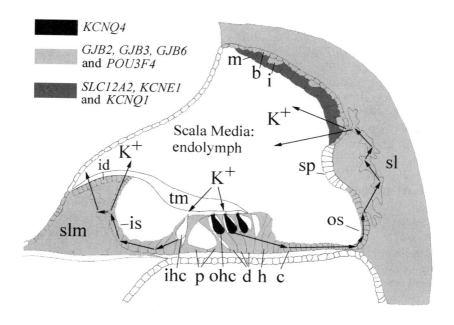

Figure 1–5. Illustration of the cochlear duct, with the proposed routes for potassium recycling indicated with arrows. Dark shading represents the expression of *KCNQ4* in outer hair cells, which may allow potassium to be removed from basolateral hair cell membranes. Pale grey regions represent the areas connected by gap junctions, thought to permit the flow of potassium back to the stria vascularis, and the gap junctional connexins encoded by *GJB2*, *GJB3*, and *GJB6* are expressed in parts of this cell network. The transcription factor gene *POU3F4* is also thought to be involved in potassium recycling by allowing extensive intercellular contacts and is expressed in the spiral ligament, among other places. The marginal cells of the stria vascularis are shaded medium gray, and these express the *SLC12A2* gene on their basolateral surfaces and the *KCNQ1* and *KCNE1* genes on their lumenal surfaces; the cotransporter encoded by *SLC12A2* participates in potassium pumping into the marginal cell, while the products of the *KCNQ1* and *KCNE1* genes together form a channel through which potassium can flow into the endolymph, restoring the high potassium concentration there. (ihc, inner hair cells; ohc, outer hair cells; p, pillar cells; d, Deiter's cells; h, Hensen's cells; c, Claudius cells; os, outer spiral sulcus cells; sp, spiral prominence; sl, spiral limbus; b, basal cells of stria vascularis; i, intermediate [melanocyte-like] cells of the stria vascularis; m, marginal cells of the stria vascularis; id, interdental cells; tm, tectorial membrane; slm, spiral limbus; is, inner sulcus cells.) (Adapted with permission from "Genes Involved in Deafness," by R. H. Holmes and K. P. Steel, 1999. *Current Opinion in Genetics and Development, 9*, 304–314. Figure prepared by Sarah Holme and Ralph Holme.)

known, but whatever their function is, it does not appear necessary for the secretion of some sort of endolymph, because there is an open scala media and no collapse of Reissner's membrane in the mutants. Other mouse mutants (and other animals with deafness and white spotting of the coat) have a similar pigmentation defect, due to a lack of melanocytes, so may also have reduced or absent endocochlear potentials, but such measurements have not yet been reported (see Steel, 1995, for a review).

As mentioned above, a number of deafness genes have recently been identified, in both human and mouse, that appear to function directly in potassium recycling in the cochlear duct (for review, see Holt & Corey, 1999; Steel, 1999; Steel & Bussoli, 1999) (see Figure 1–5). KCNQ4 encodes a potassium channel expressed in outer hair cells and is thought to be involved in removing potassium from the cells via their basolateral membranes (Kubisch et al., 1999); the gene is mutated in a form of autosomal dominant deafness in humans. From here the potassium is believed to pass through an extensive network of gap junctions between the supporting cells of the organ of Corti and the fibrocytes forming the spiral ligament on the lateral wall, back to the stria vascularis (Figure 1–5). At least three connexin genes involved in forming these gap junctions have been found to be mutated in different types of human genetic deafness. These include the *GJB2* gene, encoding connexin 26, mutated in both recessive and dominant forms of nonsyndromic deafness; the GJB3 gene, encoding connexin 31, mutated in dominant nonsyndromic deafness; and the GJB6 gene, encoding the connexin 30 molecule, which has most recently been reported to underlie another type of dominant nonsyndromic deafness (Denoyelle et al., 1998; Grifa et al., 1999; Kelsell et al., 1997; Xia et al., 1999).

The *Pou3f4* mouse mutant, with a targeted deletion of the gene, provides evidence that this gene is involved in some aspect of potassium recycling, although the mouse has a reduced endocochlear potential and no collapse of scala media, suggesting that endolymph secretion can still be maintained in the mutant (Minowa et al., 1999). The only ultrastructural defect reported was a reduction in the intercellular contacts between adjacent fibrocytes in the spiral ligament on the lateral wall, corresponding to the site of expression of this transcription factor, which is restricted to mesenchymal cells around the inner ear, including the spiral ligament fibrocytes. It is possible that these restricted contacts inhibit potassium recycling to some extent.

Having reached the stria, the potassium is pumped into the marginal cells across their basolateral membranes by a Na-K-ATPase acting in concert with a Na-K-Cl cotransporter (e.g., Wangemann, 1995). This cotransporter has recently been identified as the product of the *Slc12a2* gene, because this gene was found to be mutated in two alleles at the shaker-with-syndactylism (*sy*) locus; in the original *sy* mutation, the gene is completely deleted, and in the *sy^{ns}* allele, there is an insertion of an additional adenine in a string of six adenine bases, leading to a frameshift and premature termination codon (Dixon et al., 1999). We found in the *sy^ns* mutant, as previously reported for the *sy* mutant (Deol, 1963), that there is extensive collapse of Reissner's membrane and the walls of the vestibular compartments of the inner ear, suggesting that there is complete failure of endolymph secretion (Dixon et al., 1999). A knockout of the same gene has also been reported with the same collapse of endolymphatic compartments (Delpire, Lu, England, Dull, & Thorne, 1999).

Finally, the KCNQ1 (KvLQT1) and KCNE1 (ISK) genes are both involved in forming a potassium channel at the lumenal surface of the marginal cells, which allows the potassium pumped into the cell to flow out, down its electrochemical gradient, into the endolymph, restoring the potassium concentration there. Both genes have been found to be mutated in different families with Jervell and Lange-Nielsen syndrome (Neyroud et al., 1997; Schultze-Bahr et al., 1997). In the mouse mutant with the *Isk* gene inactivated, there is a failure of endolymph secretion and collapse of Reissner's membrane (Vetter et al., 1996).

In addition to the genes involved in potassium recycling, two other genes are likely to be involved in maintaining endolymphatic homeostasis. The pendrin gene (PDS) is mutated in Pendred syndrome and some cases of nonsyndromic deafness; it is expressed in a small group of epithelial cells just below the stria vascularis (spiral prominence and outer sulcus region), and the gene is believed to be involved in iodide and chloride transport (Everett, Morsli, Wu, & Green, 1999). Another gene, ATP6B1 encoding the B1 subunit of the H^+-ATPase proton pump, is probably involved in adjusting the pH of the endolymph by pumping hydrogen ions into scala media; this gene is expressed in the interdental cells, on the upper surface of the spiral limbus just below the attachment of the tectorial membrane, and mutations in humans cause renal tubular acidosis with deafness (Karet et al., 1999).

The number of genes now known to be involved in controlling ionic homeostasis within the cochlear duct and known to be vital for normal auditory function does suggest that this is an aspect of cochlear function that needs careful study. In particular, the finding that one of the genes, the GJB2 gene encoding connexin 26, is quite frequently involved in nonsyndromic deafness in the human population suggests that this will become a much more active area of research in the future.

MOVING FORWARD

All areas of genetic research are moving forward very rapidly, and the imminent release of extensive sequence of the human genome will revolutionize progress. However, identifying the function of genes discovered by sequence analysis will still require much empirical laboratory work. A number of deafness genes have been found by targeted knockout by groups interested in a particular gene family, but many others have been identified by starting with a mutant mouse (or human) and identifying the gene by positional cloning. The advantage of the latter approach is that you know before starting whether there is a phenotype (deafness) that is of interest to you, although the disadvantage is that positional cloning still represents a considerable effort. However, positional cloning in the mouse is still somewhat easier than positional cloning of human deafness genes. Having identified a mouse deafness gene, it is a relatively straightforward step to clone the orthologous human gene and search for mutations in it in deaf humans.

A limiting factor in our progress in identifying deafness genes is the fact that there is a gap between the number of mouse mutants that we would expect to find and the number available. This may be because mouse mutants with deafness alone would not normally be detected by animal handlers, so new deaf mutants are likely to be lost. We know these mutants are missing because when we compare the locations of the known deafness genes in the human genome with the corresponding regions of the mouse genome, there are many cases where there is no potential deaf mouse model mapping to the appropriate chromosomal region. Equally, there are many deaf mouse mutants for which no human equivalent has yet been found, such as the *Myo6* mutation described earlier.

One way forward that we have adopted is to generate many more deaf mouse mutants by a programme of random mutagenesis. Male mice are injected with a powerful mutagen, *N*-ethyl-*N*-nitrosourea (ENU), mated to normal females, and the offspring screened for new dominant mutations. The new deaf mutants are detected by their failure to respond with an ear flick (Preyer reflex) to a brief, high-frequency toneburst. New mutants with balance defects are picked up by their characteristic hyperactive, head-tossing, and/or circling behavior, and these often have hearing impairment in addition to their vestibular dysfunction. This approach has been successful in producing many new mutants, some with completely new phenotypes, and we are localizing the mutations as well as characterizing the auditory defects in them all. We anticipate that some of these at least should provide models for known human forms of genetic deafness, and facilitate the search for the responsible gene.

Having mouse models for each form of human deafness will allow us to make progress in understanding the underlying pathological processes at a molecular and cellular level, and it is only when we have this understanding that we can devise ways of treating this most common form of sensory impairment in our population.

Acknowledgments: KPS would like to thank the many collaborators, in Nottingham and around the world, who have worked with her over the years, and helped to develop the ideas and expertise we now have in our studies of deaf mouse mutants. However, she would also like to take this opportunity to thank several other people who have made important contributions in shaping the direction of her work: Mr Savory and Mr Rix, the teachers who first introduced her to biology at school; Dorothy Hodgkin, whose lecture to sixth-form school students about solving the insulin structure provided much early inspiration; Malkiat Deol, her Ph.D. advisor, who first introduced her to deaf mouse mutants; Bill Kimberling, whose sheer enthusiasm first persuaded her that identifying deafness genes was worthwhile; and Steve Brown, who agreed to help. KPS is supported by the MRC, Defeating Deafness, and the European Commission (Contracts BMH4-CT96-1324 and CT97-2715).

This chapter is dedicated to the memory of Professor Malkiat S. Deol, who died in June 1999.

REFERENCES

Avraham, K. B., Hasson, T., Sobe, T., Balsara, B., Testa, J. R., Skvorak, A. B., Morton, C. C., Copeland, N. G., & Jenkins, N. A. (1997). Characterisation of unconventional *MYO6*, the human homologue of the gene responsible for deafness in Snell's waltzer mice. *Human Molecular Genetics, 6*, 1225–1231.

Avraham, K. B., Hasson, T., Steel, K. P., Kingsley, D. M., Russell, L. B., Mooseker, M. S., Copeland, N. G., & Jenkins, N. A. (1995). The mouse *Snell's waltzer* deafness gene encodes an unconventional myosin required for structural integrity of inner hair cells. *Nature Genetics, 11*, 369–375.

Buss, F., Kendrick-Jones, J., Lionne, C., Knoght, A. E., Côté, G. P., & Luzio, J. P. (1998). The localisation of myosin VII at the Golgi complex and leading edge of fibroblasts and its phosphorylation and recruitment into membrane ruffles of A431 cells after growth factor stimulation. *Journal of Cell Biology, 143*, 1535–1545.

Bussoli, T. J., & Steel, K. P. (1999). Gene expression in the developing ear. *http://www.ihr.mrc.ac.uk/Hereditary/genetable/index.html.*

Cable, J., Huszar, D., Jaenisch, R., & Steel, K. P. (1994). Effects of mutations at the W locus (*c-kit*) on inner ear pigmentation and function in the mouse. *Pigment Cell Research, 7*, 17–32.

Cable, J., Jackson, I. J., Steel, K. P. (1993). *Light* (*B^lt^*), a mutation causing melanocyte death, leads to strial dysfunction in the inner ear. *Pigment Cell Research, 6*, 215–225.

Cable, J., Jackson, I. J. & Steel, K. P. (1995). Mutations at the W locus affect survival of neural crest-derived melanocytes in the mouse. *Mechanisms of Development, 50*, 139–150.

Cable J., & Steel, K. P. (1998). Combined cochleo-saccular and neuroepithelial abnormalities in the Varitint-waddler-J (*Va^J^*) mouse. *Hearing Research, 123*, 125–136.

Delpire, E., Lu, J., England, R., Dull, C., & Thorne, T. (1999). Deafness and imbalance associated with inactivation of the secretory Na-K-2Cl cotransporter. *Nature Genetics, 22*, 192–195.

Denoyelle, F., LinaGranade, G., Plauchu, H., Bruzzone, R., Chaib, H., LeviAcobas, F., Weil, D., & Petit, C. (1998). Connexin 26 gene linked to a dominant deafness. *Nature*, *393*, 319–320.

Denoyelle F., Marlin, S., Weil, D., Moatti, L., Chauvin, P., Garabédian, E. N., & Petit, C. (1999). Clinical features of the prevalent form of childhood deafness, DFNB1, due to a connexin-26 gene defect: Implications for genetic counselling. *Lancet*, *353*, 1298–1303.

Denoyelle, F., Weil, D., Maw, M. A., Wilcox, S. A., Lench, N. J., Allen-Powell, D. R., Osborn, A. H., Dahl, H. H. M., Middleton, A., Houseman, M. J., Dodé, C., Marlin, S., Boulila-ElGaïed, A., Grati, M., Ayadi, H., BenArab, S., Bitoun, P., Lina-Granade, G., Godet, J., Mustapha, M., Loiselet, J., El-Zir, E., Aubois, A., Joannard, A., Levilliers, J., Garabédian, E. N., Mueller, R. F., Gardner, R. J. M., & Petit, C. (1997). Prelingual deafness: High prevalence of a 30delG mutation in the connexin 26 gene. *Human Molecular Genetics*, *6*, 2173–2177.

Deol, M. S. (1956). The anatomy and development of the mutants pirouette, shaker1 and waltzer in the mouse. *Proceedings of the Royal Society London*, Ser. B, *145*, 206–213.

Deol, M. S. (1963). The development of the inner ear in mice homozygous for shaker-with-syndactylism. *Journal of Embryology and Expimental Morphology*, *11*, 493–512.

Deol, M. S., & Green, M. C. (1966). Snell's waltzer, a new mutation affecting behavior and the inner ear in the mouse. *Genetic Research Cambridge*, *8*, 339–345.

Dixon, M. J., Gazzard, J., Chaudhry, S. S., Sampson, N., Schulte, B. A., & Steel, K. P. (1999). Mutation of the basolateral Na-K-Cl cotransporter gene *Slc12a2* results in deafness in mice. *Human Molecular Genetics*, *8*, 1579–1584.

El-Amraoui, A., Sahly, I., Picaud, S., Sahel, J., Abitbol, M., & Petit, C. (1996). Human Usher 1B/mouse shaker1: The retinal phenotype discrepancy explained by presence/absence of myosin VIIA in the photoreceptor cells. *Human Molecular Genetics*, *5*, 1171–1178.

Emmerling, M. R., & Sobkowicz, H. M. (1990). Acetylcholinesterase-positive innervation in cochleas from two strains of shaker1 mice. *Hearing Research*, *47*, 25–38.

Estivill, X., Fortina, P., Surrey, S., Rabionet, R., Melchionda, S., D'Agruma, L., Mansfield, E., Rappaport, E., Govea, N., Milà, M., Zelante, L., & Gasparini, P. (1998). Connexin-26 mutations in sporadic and inherited sensorineural deafness. *Lancet*, *351*, 394–398.

Everett, L. A., Morsli, H., Wu, D. K., & Green, E. D. (1999). Expression pattern of a mouse ortholog of the Pendred's syndrome gene (*Pds*) suggests a key role for Pendrin in the inner ear. *Procedings of the National Academy of Science, USA*, *96*, 9727–9732.

Fekete, D. M. (1999). Development of the vertebrate ear: Insight from knockouts and mutants. *Trends in Neurosciences*, *22*, 263–269.

Fortnum, H., & Davis, A. (1997). Epidemiology of permanent childhood hearing impairment in Trent region, 1985-1993. *British Journal of Audiology*, *31*, 409–446.

Gibson, F., Walsh, J., Mburu, P., Varela, A., Brown, K. A., Antonio, M., Beisel, K. W., Steel, K. P., & Brown, S. D. M. (1995). A type VII myosin encoded by the mouse deafness gene *shaker-1*. *Nature*, *374*, 62–64.

Grifa, A., Wagner, C. A., D'Ambrosio, L., Melchionda, S., Bernardi, F., Lopez-Bigas, N., Rabionet, R., Arbones, M., Della Monica, M., Estivill, X., Zelante, L., Lang, F.,

& Gasparini, P. (1999). Mutations in *GJB6* cause nonsyndromic autosomal dominant deafness at DFNA3 locus. *Nature Genetics, 23,* 16–18.

Harvey, D. (1989). *Structural and functional development of the cochlea in normal (CBA/Ca) and hearing impaired shaker1 (sh1/sh1) mice* [Ph.D. thesis]. University of Nottingham, UK.

Hasson, T., Gillespie, P. G., Garcia, J. A., MacDonald, R. B., Zhao, Y., Yee, A. G., Mooseker, M. S., & Corey, D. P. (1997). Unconventional myosins in inner ear sensory epithelia. *Journal of Cell Biology, 137,* 1287–1307.

Hasson, T., Heintzelman, J., Santos-Sacchi, J., Corey, D. P., & Mooseker, M. S. (1995). Expression in cochlea and retina of myosin VIIa, the gene product defective in Usher syndrome type 1B. *Procedings of the National Academy of Science, USA, 92,* 9815–9819.

Hasson, T., Walsh, J., Cable, J., Mooseker, M. S., Brown, S. D. M., & Steel, K. P. (1997). Effects of shaker-1 mutations on myosin-VIIa protein and mRNA expression. *Cell Motility and the Cytoskeleton, 37,* 127–138.

Holme, R. H., & Steel, K. P. (1999). Genes involved in deafness. *Current Opinion in Genetics and Development, 9,* 309–314.

Holt, J. R., & Corey, D. P. (1999). Ion channel defects in hereditary hearing loss. *Neuron, 22,* 217–219.

Karet, F. E., Finberg, K. E., Nelson, R. D., Nayir, A., Mocan, H., Sanjad, S. A., Rodriguez-Soriano, J., Santos, F., Cremers, C. W. R. J., Di Pietro, A., Hoffbrand, B. I., Winiarski, J., Bakkaloglu, A., Ozen, S., Dusunsel, R., Goodyer, P., Hulten, S. A., Wu, D. K., Skvorak, A. B., Morton, C. C., Cunningham, M. J., Jha, V., & Lifton, R. P. (1999). Mutations in the gene encoding B1 subunit of H^+-ATPase cause renal tubular acidosis with sensorineural deafness. *Nature Genetics, 21,* 84–90.

Keats, B. J. B., & Berlin, C. I. (1999). Genomics and hearing impairment. *Genome Research, 9,* 7–16.

Kelley, P. M., Harris, D. J., Comer, B. C., Askew, J. W., Fowler, T., Smith, S. D., & Kimberling, W. J. (1998). Novel mutations in the connexin 26 gene (*GJB2*) that cause autosomal recessive (DFNB1) hearing loss. *American Journal of Human Genetics, 62,* 792–799.

Kelsell, D. P., Dunlop, J., Stevens, H. P., Lench, N. J., Liang, J. N., Parry, G., Mueller, R. F., & Leigh, I. M. (1997). Connexin26 mutations in hereditary nonsyndromic sensorineural deafness. *Nature, 387,* 80–83.

Kiernan, A., & Steel, K. P. (in press). Mouse homologues for human deafness. In K. Kitamura & K. P. Steel (Eds.), *Genetics in otolaryngology.* Basel, Switzerland: Karger.

Kikuchi, T., Kimura, R. S., Paul, D. L., & Adams, J. C. (1995). Gap junctions in the rat cochlea: Immunohistochemical and ultrastructural analysis. *Anatomy and Embryology, 191,* 101–118.

Kubisch, C., Schroeder, B. C., Friedrich, T., Lütjohann, B., El-Amraoui, A., Marlin, S., Petit, C., & Jentsch, T. J. (1999). KCNQ4, a novel potassium channel expressed in sensory outer hair cells, is mutated in dominant deafness. *Cell, 96,* 437–446.

Liu, X., Ondek, B., & Williams, D. S. (1998). Mutant myosin VIIa causes defective melanosome distribution in the RPE of shaker1 mice. *Nature Genetics, 19,* 117–118.

Liu, X., Udovichenko, I. P., Brown, S. D. M., Steel, K. P., & Williams, D. S. (1999). Myosin VIIa is required for normal opsin distribution in the photoreceptor cilium: Implications for blindness in Usher syndrome. *Journal of Neuroscience, 19,* 6267–6274.

Liu, X., Vansant, G., Udovichenko, I. P., Wolfrum, U., & Williams, D. S. (1997). Myosin VIIA, the product of the Usher 1B syndrome gene, is concentrated in the connecting cilia of photoreceptor cells. *Cell Motility and the Cytoskeleton, 37,* 240–252.

Liu, X.-Z., Hope, C., Walsh, J., Newton, V., Ke, X. M., Liang, C. Y., Xu, L. R., Zhou, J. M., Trump, D., Steel, K. P., Bundey, S., & Brown, S. D. M. (1998). Mutations in the myosin VIIA gene cause a wide phenotypic spectrum including atypical Usher syndrome. *American Journal of Human Genetics, 63,* 909–912.

Liu, X.-Z., Walsh, J., Mburu, P., Kendrick-Jones, J., Cope, J., Steel, K. P., & Brown, S. D. M. (1997). Mutations in the myosin VIIA gene causing nonsyndromic recessive deafness. *Nature Genetics, 16,* 188–190.

Liu, X.-Z., Walsh, J., Tamagawa, Y., Kitamura, K., Nishizawa, M., Steel, K. P., & Brown, S. D. M. (1997). Autosomal dominant nonsyndromic deafness caused by a mutation in the myosin VIIA gene. *Nature Genetics, 17,* 268–269.

Lord, E. M., & Gates, W. H. (1929). Shaker, a new mutation of the house mouse (Mus musculus). *American Naturalist, 63,* 435–442.

Mburu, P., Liu, X. Z., Walsh, J., Saw, D., Cope, J. T. V., Gibson, F., Kendrick-Jones, J., Steel, K. P., & Brown, S. D. M. (1997). Mutation analysis of the mouse myosin VIIA deafness gene—A putative myosin motor-kinesin tail hybrid. *Genes and Function, 1,* 191–203.

Mermall, V., McNally, J. G., & Miller, K. G. (1994). Transport of cytoplasmic vesicles catalysed by an unconventional myosin in living *Drosophila* embryos. *Nature, 369,* 560–562.

Mermall, V., Post, P. L., & Mooseker, M. S. (1998). Unconventional myosins in cell movement, membrane traffic, and signal transduction. *Science, 279,* 527–533.

Minowa, O., Ikeda, K., Sugitani, Y., Oshima, T., Nakai, S., Katori, Y., Suzuki, M., Furukawa, M., Kawase, T., Zheng, Y., Ogura, M., Asada, Y., Watanabe, K., Yamanaka, H., Gotoh, S., Nishi-Takeshima, M., Sugimoto, T., Kikuchi, T., Takasaka, T., & Noda, T. (1999). Altered cochlear fibrocytes in a mouse model of DFN3 nonsyndromic deafness. *Science, 285,* 1408–1411.

Morell, R. J., Kim, H. J., Hood, L. J., Goforth, L., Friderici, K., Fisher, R., Van Camp, G., Berlin, C. I., Oddoux, C., Ostrer, H., Keats, B., & Friedman, T. B. (1998). Mutations in the connexin 26 gene (*GJB2*) among Ashkenazi Jews with nonsyndromic recessive deafness. *New England Journal of Medicine, 339,* 1500–1505.

Morton, N. E. (1991). Genetic epidemiology of hearing impairment. In R. J. Ruben, T. R. Van De Water, & K. P. Steel (Eds.), Genetics of hearing impairment. *Annals of the New York Academy of Science, 630,* 16–31.

Neyroud, N., Tesson, F., Denjoy, I., Leibovici, M., Donger, C., Barhanin, J., Faure, S., Gary, F., Coumel, P., Petit, C., Schwartz, K., & Guicheney, P. (1997). A novel mutation in the potassium channel gene KVLQT1 causes the Jervell and Lange-Nielsen cardioauditory syndrome. *Nature Genetics, 15,* 186–189.

Online Mendelian Inheritance in Man, OMIM™ Center for Medical Genetics, Johns Hopkins University (Baltimore, MD) and National Center for Biotechnology Information, National Library of Medicine (Bethesda, MD), (1999). World Wide Web URL: *http://www.ncbi.nlm.nih.gov/Omim*

Probst, F. J., & Camper, S. A. (1999). The role of mouse mutants in the identification of human hereditary hearing loss genes. *Hearing Research, 130,* 1–6.

Probst, F. J., Fridell, R. A., Raphael, Y., Saunders, T. L., Wang, A., Liang, Y., Morell, R. J., Touchman, J. W., Lyons, R. H., Noben-Trauth, K., Friedman, T. B., & Camper, S. A. (1998). Correction of deafness in shaker2 mice by an unconventional myosin in a BAC transgene. *Science, 280,* 1444–1447.

Richardson, G. P., Forge, A., Kros, C. J., Fleming, J., Brown, S. D. M., & Steel, K. P. (1997). Myosin VIIA is required for aminoglycoside accumulation in cochlear hair cells. *Journal of Neuroscience, 17,* 9506–9519.

Schuknecht, H. F. (1974). *Pathology of the ear.* Cambridge, MA: Harvard University Press.

Schulze-Bahr, E., Wang, Q., Wedekind, H., Haverkamp, W., Chen, Q. Y., Sun, Y. L., Rubie, C., Hordt, M., Towbin, J. A., Borggrefe, M., Assmann, G., Qu, X. D., Somberg, J. C., Breithardt, G., Oberti, C., & Funke, H. (1997). *KCNE1* mutations cause Jervell and Lange-Nielsen syndrome. *Nature Genetics, 17,* 267–268.

Self, T., Mahony, M., Fleming, J., Walsh, J., Brown, S. D. M., & Steel, K. P. (1998). Shaker-1 mutations reveal roles for myosin VIIA in both development and function of cochlear hair cells. *Development, 125,* 557–566.

Self, T., Sobe, T., Copeland, N. G., Jenkins, N. A., Avraham, K. B., & Steel, K. P. (1999). Role of myosin VI in the development of cochlear hair cells. *Developmental Biology, 214,* 331–341.

Spicer, S. S., & Schulte, B. A. (1996). The fine structure of spiral ligament cells relates to ion return to the stria and varies with place-frequency. *Hearing Research, 100,* 80–100.

Steel, K. P. (1995). Inherited hearing defects in mice. *Annual Review of Genetics, 29,* 675–701.

Steel, K. P. (1998a). A new era in the genetics of deafness. *New England Journal of Medicine, 339,* 1545–1547.

Steel, K. P. (1998b). Progress in progressive deafness. *Science, 279,* 1870–1871.

Steel, K. P. (1999). The benefits of recycling. *Science, 285,* 1363–1364.

Steel, K. P., & Barkway, C. (1989). Another role for melanocytes: Their importance for normal stria vascularis development in the mammalian inner ear. *Development, 107,* 453–463.

Steel, K. P., Barkway, C., & Bock, G. R. (1987). Strial dysfunction in mice with cochleo-saccular abnormalities. *Hearing Research, 27,* 11–26.

Steel, K. P., & Bock, G. R. (1983). Hereditary inner ear abnormalities in animals. Relationships with human abnormalities. *Archives of Otolaryngology, 109,* 22–29.

Steel, K. P., & Bussoli, T. J. (1999). Deafness genes: Expressions of surprise. *Trends in Genetics, 15,* 207–211.

Steel, K. P., Davidson, D. R., & Jackson, I. J. (1992). TRP-2/DT, a new early melanoblast marker, shows that steel growth factor (c-kit ligand) is a survival factor. *Development, 115,* 1111–1119.

Steel, K. P., & Harvey, D. (1992). Development of auditory function in mutant mice. In R. Romand (Ed.), *Development of audiology and vestibular systems* (Vol. 2, pp. 221–242). Amsterdam: Elsevier Press.

Steel, K. P., & Smith, R. J. H. (1992). Normal hearing in *splotch* (*Sp*/+), the mouse homologue of Waardenburg syndrome type 1. *Nature Genetics, 2,* 75–79.

Suga, F., & Hattler, K. W. (1970). Physiological and histopathological correlates of hereditary deafness in animals. *Laryngoscope, 80,* 81–104.

Van Camp, G., & Smith, R. J. H. (1999). *Hereditary hearing loss homepage.* Available: World Wide Web URL: *http://dnalab-www.uia.ac.be/dnalab/hhh/*

Vetter, D. E., Mann, J. R., Wangemann, P., Liu, J. Z., McLaughlin, K. J., Lesage, F., Marcus, D. C., Lazdunski, M., Heinemann, S.F., & Barhanin, J. (1996). Inner ear defects induced by null mutation of the *isk* gene. *Neuron, 17,* 1251–1264.

Wang, A., Liang, Y., Fridell, R. A., Probst, F. J., Wilcox, E. R., Touchman, J. W., Morton, C. C., Morell, R. J., Noben-Trauth, K., Camper, S. A., & Friedman, T. B. (1998). Association of unconventional myosin *MYO15* mutations with human nonsyndromic deafness *DFNB3*. *Science, 280,* 1447–1451.

Wangemann, P. (1995). Comparison of ion transport mechanisms between vestibular dark cells and strial marginal cells. *Hearing Research, 90,* 149–157.

Weil, D., Blanchard, S., Kaplan, J., Guilford, P., Gibson, F., Walsh, J., Mburu, P., Varela, A., Levilliers, J., Weston, M. D., Kelley, P. M., Kimberling, W. J., Wagenaar, M., Levi-Acobas, F., Larget-Piet, D., Munnich, A., Steel, K. P., Brown, S. D. M., & Petit, C. (1995). Defective myosin VIIA gene responsible for Usher syndrome type 1B. *Nature, 374,* 60–61.

Weil, D., Küssel, P., Blanchard, S., Lévy, G., Levi-Acobas, F., Drira, M., Ayadi, H., & Petit, C. (1997). The autosomal recessive isolated deafness, DFNB2, and the Usher 1B syndrome are allelic defects of the myosin VIIA gene. *Nature Genetics, 16,* 191–193.

Wells, A. L., Lin, A., Chen, L. Q., Safer, D., Cain, S. M., Hasson, T., Carraghers, B. O., Milligan, R. A., & Sweeney, H. L. (1999). Myosin VI is an actin-based motor that moves backwards. *Nature, 401,* 505–508.

Xia, J. H., Liu, C. Y., Tang, B. S., Pan, Q., Huang, L., Dai, H. P., Zhang, B. R., Xie, W., Hu, D. X., Zheng, D., Shi, X. L., Wang, D. A., Xia, K., Yu, K. P., Liao, X. D., Feng, Y., Yang, Y. F., Xiao, J. Y., Xie, D. H., & Huang, J. Z. (1998). Mutations in the gene encoding gap junction protein beta-3 associated with autosomal dominant hearing impairment. *Nature Genetics, 20,* 370–373.

Zelante, L., Gasparini, P., Estivill, X., Melchionda, S., D'Agruma, L., Govea, N., Milá, M., Della Monica, M., Lutfi, J., Shohat, M., Mansfield, E., Delgrosso, K., Rappaport, E., Surrey, S., & Fortina, P. (1997). Connexin26 mutations associated with the most common form of nonsyndromic deafness (DFNB1) in Mediterraneans. *Human Molecular Genetics, 6,* 1605–1609.

2

The Myosin-15 Molecular Motor is Necessary for Hearing in Humans and Mice: A Review of DFNB3 and *shaker-2*

Thomas B. Friedman, Frank J. Probst, Edward R. Wilcox,
John T. Hinnant, Yong Liang, Aihui Wang, Thomas D. Barber,
Anil K. Lalwani, David W. Anderson, I. Nyoman Arhya,
Sunaryana Winata, Sukarti Moeljapowiro, James H. Asher, Jr.,
David Dolan, Yehoash Raphael, Robert A. Fridell, Sally A. Camper

In the early 1990s, several research groups realized independently that the genetic, molecular, and conceptual tools were finally available to effectively map and identify mouse and human genes for hereditary hearing impairment. In mice, many mutated genes causing hearing loss phenotypes were available, and some were likely to be orthologues of defective genes that cause deafness in humans (Steel, 1995). Identifying mouse genes for deafness was bound to give insight into mammalian auditory function in general, a long-held, prescient viewpoint of Dr. Karen Steel. A particular strength of the mouse as a model system is that the number of parent to offspring transmissions can be very large, permitting the responsible genes to be rapidly mapped to a small chromosomal interval. Moreover, the mouse and human auditory systems are very similar.

In contrast to mice, a genetic analysis of human hereditary hearing impairment requires identification of multigenerational families or an isolated population containing several hearing-impaired individuals. Hereditary deafness in humans is one of the most common neurosensory deficits, so ascertaining small families is straightforward, but they often do not help in mapping genes. Despite this obstacle, over 60 genes for nonsyndromic deafness have now been mapped, and many more remain to be discovered.

This chapter describes the novel experimental strategies used to identify DFNB3, the third human gene for hereditary nonsyndromic recessive deafness to be mapped. The story begins in Bengkala, Bali, Indonesia, a village in a rural farming area where there are 48 profoundly deaf individuals (Figure 2–1A). Bengkala is an old village, as evidenced by metallic plaques (*prasasti*) from 1178 AD commemorating its incorporation. In 1992, the large proportion of deaf individuals (2.2%) living in Bengkala was brought to the attention of the late Dr. James H. Asher, Jr. by two Indonesian academic physicians, I. Nyoman Arhya and Sunaryana Winata. Jim was teaching a human genetics course in Indonesia. Sunaryana was in attendance and mentioned Bengkala to Jim, prompting a visit by them to Bengkala that year. Thus began a 6-year project to identify the gene responsible for hereditary deafness in this village, as well as anthropological and linguistic studies of the people of Bengkala. The next year a few of us began an interdisciplinary investigation of hereditary deafness in this village.

The deaf individuals of Bengkala use a unique sign language that is understood by most of the 2254 members of the hearing population of the village. In the next chapter, details of the social lives of the people of Bengkala and their sign language are described as well as being illustrated on the CD-ROM accompanying this book.

DEAFNESS IN BENGKALA IS CONGENITAL AND PROFOUND

The deaf population of Bengkala is one of a few examples of a relatively large group of deaf people who are well integrated into their local community. The hearing and deaf residents live in residential clusters based on descent from common male ancestors. Babies born to deaf parents are checked immediately and periodically thereafter for signs of deafness by clapping hands, beating on water buckets, or gamelan orchestra cymbals. A child is considered deaf if there is no startle response to the loud noise. Deaf and hearing children are socialized together, and learn the unique Bengkala sign language from one another. Before hearing children are able to speak fluently they have been seen signing with their deaf playmates.

There are currently 24 deaf males and 24 deaf females in Bengkala. Some hearing parents from Bengkala have both hearing and deaf children. Seventeen congenitally deaf individuals in Bengkala have two hearing parents. When both parents are deaf, with one exception, all of the children are born profoundly deaf (Figure 2–1A). The explanation is genetic complementation. When a deaf person from Bengkala marries a deaf person from another village, they often have hearing children, suggesting that the deafness segregating in most of the other nearby Balinese villages is not due to mutations at the DFNB3 locus.

Given what we know about the hereditary deafness in Bengkala, the most parsimonious explanation for this pattern of inheritance is an autosomal recessive mutation of a single gene (Winata et al., 1995). Fortuitously, as we began to gather clinical data on deafness in Bengkala and to initiate an effort to map the responsible gene, we discovered several consanguineous families living in India with congenital deafness linked to DFNB3. We also found a genetic link to a deaf strain of mice known as *shaker-2*.

DFNB3 Maps to Chromosome 17 at p11.2

Over many generations the mutation causing deafness in Bengkala has been disseminated among many of the villagers. Assortative mating, the preference of deaf individuals for deaf spouses, has also increased the number of deaf individuals in Bengkala. Approximately 2.2% of the people of Bengkala are congenitally deaf. Other such communities with a high proportion of hereditary deafness have been described (Groce, 1985; Shuman, 1980). The molecular basis of the hearing loss is now known for the village of Adamarobe, Ghana (a mutation of GJB2, connexin 26) (Brobby, Muller-Myhsok, & Horstmann, 1998) and for Bengkala, Bali (Wang et al., 1998).

In isolated populations and in consanguineous families, affected individuals with recessively inherited diseases most likely carry two copies of the same mutation. That is, they are homozygous by descent for the same mutant allele of DFNB3. Based on this assumption, the strategy we used to map DFNB3 was to identify, via a genome wide screen, a region of homozygosity in all affected individuals from Bengkala. Homozygosity mapping was proposed as a strategy decades ago but has only recently been popularized (Kruglyak, Daly, & Lander, 1995; Lander & Botstein, 1987; Smith, 1953) and is now frequently used to refine the map positions of genes (Aksentijevich et al., 1993; Ben Hamida et al., 1993; Pollak et al., 1993).

DNA samples were obtained from deaf and hearing people of Bengkala in June 1993. That fall, in the laboratory of Dr. James Weber at the Marshfield Medical Research Foundation, two of us (TBF and YL) mapped DFNB3 to a 12 cM interval of the pericentromeric region of chromosome 17 (Friedman et al., 1995). Further work refined DFNB3 to a 4-5 centiMorgan (cM) region of the short arm (p) of chromosome 17 in band 11.2 (Liang et al., 1998). The 17p11.2 region is rich in genes, with a daunting number of good DFNB3 candidates (Liang et al., 1998). One gene adjacent to the DFNB3 critical region is PMP22. A duplication or point mutations of

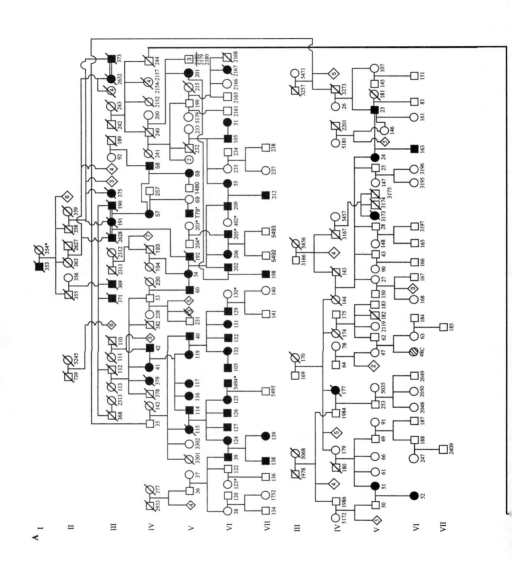

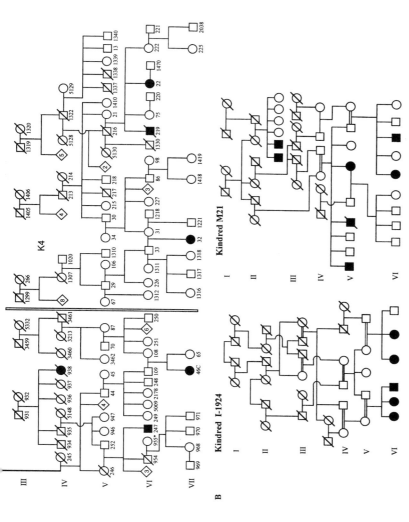

Figure 2–1. A. Partial genealogy of families with deaf individuals from Bengkala, Bali (Liang et al., 1998). Blackened symbols represent congenitally deaf individuals. The hatched symbol (individual 48C) denotes deafness that likely was acquired and not genetic since this individual is not homozygous for or even carrying a MYO15 mutation. According to her relatives, individual 48C lost her hearing in childhood. An asterisk indicates an individual living in Bengkala but originating from another Balinese village. **B.** Two consanguineous Indian families, I-1924 and M-21, with profound congenital deafness linked to DFNB3, have mutations in MYO15 (Figure modified from Liang et al., 1998).

35

PMP22 cause Charcot-Marie Tooth disease. *Pmp22*, the mouse ortholog of PMP22, is on mouse chromosome 11. Very near *Pmp22* on chromosome 11 is the *shaker-2* locus. Like humans homozygous for DFNB3, *shaker-2* mice are profoundly deaf due to a recessive mutation (Dobrovolskaia-Zavasd-kaia, 1928). We hypothesized that *shaker-2* and DFNB3 are orthologous genes. At the University of Michigan's Department of Human Genetics, two of us (SC and FP) began an effort to rapidly clone the *shaker-2* locus as the remainder of the team worked to further refine the map position of DFNB3.

DFNB3 Families in India

Genotyping additional DFNB3 families might reveal recombinant chromosomes that would permit refinement of the DFNB3 region, thus reducing the number of DFNB3 candidate genes that would have to be screened for mutations. Additional DFNB3 families would also help demonstrate a causal connection between a putative DFNB3 mutation and deafness in each DFNB3 family. As we were refining the map position of DFNB3, two of us (EW and AL) and our research colleagues from the district of Kolhapur, Maharashtra State, India were ascertaining consanguineous families from India with profound nonsyndromic recessive deafness. The deafness segregating two of these families (Figure 2–1B) proved to be linked to genetic markers in the 17p11.2 region. These families were crucial in establishing a causal connection between mutations of a candidate DFNB3 gene and the deafness segregating in these families (Liang et al., 1998; Wang et al., 1998).

Functional Cloning of *shaker-2*, the Mouse Homologue of DFNB3

The phenotype of *shaker-2* mice includes circling behavior and profound deafness. The circling and head-tossing behavior of *shaker-2* mice is indicative of a severe vestibular defect. The *shaker-2* gene was mapped in a 500 meiosis mouse cross, providing a resolution of 0.2 cM on chromosome 11 (~400 to 800 kilobase pairs (kb) of DNA). Because of the conserved synteny between mouse chromosome 11 and human chromosome 17, we were able to utilize markers for human genes from the corresponding human gene map (Liang et al., 1998; Wang et al., 1998) to refine the mouse genetic map. Several mouse YACs (*y*east *a*rtificial *c*hromosomes) and BACs (*b*acterial *a*rtificial *c*hromosomes) carrying the genomic DNA that span the *shaker-2* region were identified. The next step usually undertaken in this sort of effort is to screen all of the BACs for genes with a mutation responsible for the *shaker-2* phenotype. However, these methods are labor intensive, especially when applied to large genomic regions. To clone *shaker-2* expeditiously we employed a strategy involving "gene rescue" coupled with large scale DNA sequencing (Probst et al., 1998). BACs from the *shaker-2* region were injected into the pronuclei of homozygous *shaker-2* fertilized eggs. These eggs were then transferred to wild type foster mothers. In doing this experiment, we hoped to recover a transgenic *shaker-2* mouse with normal hearing and no circling behavior. Would a BAC containing the entire *shaker-2* gene correct the deafness and circling behavior of *shaker-2* even if the BAC was integrated into a chromosomal site other than the normal location (ectopic site) of the *shaker-2* gene on chromosome 11?

The first BAC from the *shaker-2* critical region that we began injecting into fertilized eggs was BAC425p24. Remarkably, one transgenic *shaker-2* homozygous mouse injected with this BAC was born that did not circle and exhibited a startle response to sound. This mouse, named Sebastian, was mated with several *shaker-2* females. Approximately half of Sebastian's offspring could hear. DNA analysis confirmed that all of the hearing offspring inherited BAC425p24 while all of the deaf offspring did not (i.e. nontransgenic *shaker-2* mice). The location of *shaker-2* was now refined from ~400–800 kb on chromosome 11 to just the 140 kb of DNA contained in BAC425p24. The NIH Intramural Sequencing Center and SeqWright (Houston, TX) determined the DNA sequence of most of BAC425p24. Analysis of the sequence of this BAC predicted the presence of two genes. The first is the mouse ortholog of a previously described human GTP-binding protein gene, *Drg2* (Schenker, Lach, Kessler, Calderara, & Trueb, 1994). We sequenced the coding region of this gene in DFNB3 probands and found no mutations in deaf individuals from Bengkala or from the two DFNB3 Indian families. The second gene predicted to reside on BAC425p24 is a novel unconventional myosin, which was named *Myo15*. The human orthologue was named MYO15.

Myosins are motor-proteins that bind cytoskeletal actin and hydrolyze ATP to produce force and unidirectional movement on actin. There are many different types of myosin heavy chain genes in fungi, plants, and animal cells (Mermall, Post, & Mooseker, 1998). Myosin genes have an evolutionarily conserved motor domain at the amino terminus and a C-terminal tail domain that is divergent between myosin classes (Figure 2–2). Myosin genes are subdivided into conventional myosins (myosin class II of muscle and nonmuscle cells) and unconventional myosins (classes I and III–XV) (Mermall et al., 1998; Wang et al., 1998).

There is precedent for mutations in unconventional myosin genes causing both dominant and recessive nonsyndromic deafness. Mutations of *Myo6* cause deafness in mice (Avraham et al., 1995) and mutations of MYO7A cause dominant and recessive nonsyndromic deafness (DFNA11 and DFNB2) as well as Usher syndrome type 1B in humans (Adato et al., 1997; Liu et al., 1997; Mburu et al., 1997; Weil et al., 1995). In general, unconventional myosins have a role in intracellular transport of cargo such as specific proteins, RNA, and organelles and are involved in the processes

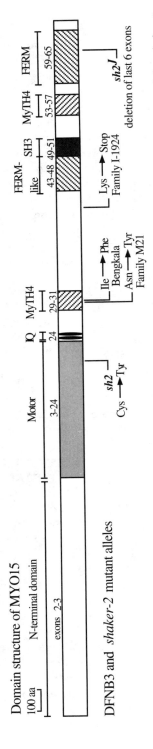

Figure 2–2. MYO15 domain structure, three mutations associated with human nonsyndromic recessive deafness *DFNB3* and the *shaker-2* mutation. The length of the longest MYO15 transcript assembled from overlapping cDNA clones is ~11.8 kb. The myosin-15 protein comprises 3530 amino acids with a predicted molecular weight of ~395 kD. Like all myosins, myosin-15 has a highly conserved motor domain. Downstream that contains an actin and an ATP binding sites. Upstream of the motor domain is a novel 1223 amino acid N-terminal domain. Downstream of the motor domain are two IQ motifs that are predicted to interact with calmodulin or related calcium binding proteins. Based on similarity to regions observed in other proteins, several functional domains are recognizable within the myosin-15 tail. These include a protein interaction motif of the src-homology 3 (SH3) class, two myosin-tail-homology 4 (MyTH4) domains and at least one FERM domain (also referred to as a band 4.1 superfamily homology domain or talin motif) (Chishti et al., 1998). Additional similarity with other proteins was observed in the region encoded by exons 43 to 48. There is an ~100 amino acid-long sequence that is similar to an internal sequence of the first FERM domain of class VII myosins. But this sequence was not recognized as a FERM domain by a ProfileScan search. The numbers in the diagram indicate the exon(s) of MYO15 encoding the domain or motif.

of endocytosis, regulating ion channels, localizing calmodulin, and cross-linking extensions of filopodia (Baker & Titus, 1998; Mermall et al., 1998; Titus, 1998). However, the precise roles of *Myo6*, MYO7A and MYO15 in the hearing process are unknown.

The genomic structure of mouse *Myo15* and human MYO15 is now known and consists of 66 exons (Liang et al., 1999), 16 more than were identified than when Wang and co-workers (1998) first reported the partial sequence of this gene (Figure 2–2). The sequence of mouse *Myo15* allowed us to screen for the mutations responsible for the *shaker-2* phenotype. In *shaker-2* mice a single nucleotide change was found in codon 1779 within exon 20. This G to A transition mutation in the motor domain of myosin-15 results in a cysteine to tyrosine substitution. The vast majority of all conventional and unconventional myosins have a cysteine at this position (http://www.mrc-lmb.cam.ac.uk/myosin/myosin.html) (Cope, Whisstock, Rayment, & Kendrick-Jones, 1996). Additionally, a second allele of *shaker-2*, *shaker-2J*, was discovered at the Jackson Laboratory in 1993 (Cook & Davisson, 1993). Like the original *shaker-2* mice, *shaker-2J* mice are profoundly deaf and exhibit circling behavior. Molecular genetic analysis has demonstrated that *shaker-2J* mice have a deletion that removes the last six exons and the polyadenylation signal of the *Myo15* gene (Anderson et al., submitted).

Myo15 is Expressed in the Sensory Organs of the Inner Ear

The location of *Myo15* mRNA expression was determined by in-situ hybridization of paraffin sections of 17.5-day post coitum wild type (C57BL/6J) mouse embryos (Figure 2–3). The tissue was hybridized with an anti-sense radiolabeled riboprobe specific for exons 48 to 51 in the tail region of *Myo15*. The results demonstrate that *Myo15* has a limited distribution to discrete patches of the cochlea, the saccule, and the utricle consistent with the positions of the sensory epithelium. The localization of *Myo15* to these sensory organs provides further evidence that the mutations discovered in *Myo15* are responsible for the phenotypes observed in *shaker-2* and *shaker-2J* mice.

Mutations of Human MYO15 Cause Deafness

The sequence of the *Myo15* gene was used to isolate the human MYO15 gene (Wang et al., 1998). Three human genomic cosmid clones containing MYO15 were isolated and 90 kb of DNA was sequenced. Predicted human MYO15 exons were identified and confirmed by sequencing human MYO15 cDNA synthesized from human fetal inner ear mRNA (generously provided by Dr. C. Morton) and from fetal brain and adult pituitary gland mRNA. MYO15 DNA was also sequenced from probands of the three

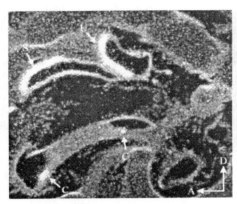 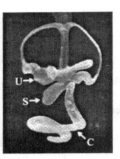

Figure 2–3. In-situ hybridization of a *Myo15* probe to 17.5 day embryonic mouse inner ear. The sections were prepared by fixing the heads in 4% paraformaldehyde and embedding them in paraffin, which was then cut at 10 micrometers in the sagittal plane and hybridized with a radiolabeled anti-sense riboprobe specific for exons 48 to 51 of the *Myo15* cDNA. The results were visualized by coating the tissue with a thin layer of photographic emulsion. The emulsion was exposed for one week, then developed and fixed. The section on the left was photographed in dark field. The section is oriented with anterior (A) to the left and dorsal (D) towards the top. In the inner ear, *Myo15* mRNA is localized in the utricle (U), saccule (S), and cochlea (C). The section was examined under high magnification by bright field microscopy. The regions indicated by the arrows contain a high density of grains in the photographic emulsion. The other bright areas lack any appreciable quantity of grains and are due instead to the presence of pigments or the refractivity of the tissue. There was no signal observed when the corresponding sense riboprobe was used. The image to the right is a paint-filled 17-day embryonic mouse inner ear (courtesy of Dr. Doris K. Wu) that is used to indicate the corresponding structures referred to in the tissue section.

DFNB3 families to identify the human MYO15 mutations that cause deafness. Mutations in MYO15 were found which co-segregated with deafness in each of the three DFNB3 families (Wang et al., 1998) (Figure 2–2). The mutations of MYO15 in Bengkala villagers and in the M-21 Indian family result in single amino acid substitutions within the first of two myosin-tail-homology 4 domains (MyTH4). This domain is similar in amino acid sequence to regions found in some other unconventional myosins including human MYO7A, *C. elegans Myo12*, bovine myosin-X and Acanthamoeba HMW myosin-IV. The function of the MyTh4 domain is unknown (Mermall et al., 1998). The mutation segregating in the Indian family I-1924 introduces a nonsense mutation which truncates the MYO15 open reading frame, resulting in either a foreshortened protein or none at all (Wang et al., 1998).

Hair Cell Stereocilia of *shaker-2* Are Abnormally Short

Light and electron microscopic examination of the hair cells of the cochlea of wild type mice and *shaker-2* and *shaker-2J* mice was undertaken (Figure 2–4). The inner ear tissue from these mice was dissected from the bony cochlea, the tectorial membrane was removed, and the remaining tissue, which contained the inner hair cells, outer hair cells and supporting cells, was examined. The hair cells were present in both *shaker-2* and *shaker-2J*, but the stereocilia on the inner and outer hair cells were very short, approximately one tenth the normal length. In addition, using rhodamine-conjugated phalloidin, we also detected abnormally thick actin bundles within the inner hair cell cytoplasm.

The stereocilia of the inner hair cells are essential for sensing the sound pressure applied to the fluid in the cochlea. The short stereocilia in both *shaker-2* and *shaker-2J* may explain the lack of hearing in these mice. So far, histopathology of the inner ear of an individual homozygous for a DFNB3 mutation has not been possible. It may well be that humans homozygous for MYO15 mutations also have shortened stereocilia just as we see in *shaker-2*.

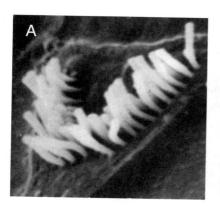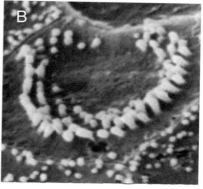

Figure 2–4. The stereocilia of *shaker-2* mutants are abnormally short. The stereocilia on a single outer hair cell from the cochlea of a normal mouse (left panel) shows long stereocilia arranged in a V-shaped array. A comparable outer hair cell from a *shaker-2* mutant (right panel) has stereocilia arranged in the typical pattern, but these stereocilia are markedly reduced in size (~7500× magnification in both panels).

EPIDEMIOLOGY OF DFNB3

Once the mutation in MYO15 segregating in Bengkala was identified, it became possible to determine the carrier frequency of this mutation among hearing individuals from Bengkala who have no known deaf relatives. In an earlier paper (Friedman et al., 1995) we referred to these individuals as representative Bengkala individuals (RBIs). Of a sample of 48 RBIs, we discovered that the DFNB3 mutation is carried by 25%. This is higher than the predicted carrier rate for DFNB3 of 17.2% made by Winata and co-workers before DFNB3 was cloned and before we could directly determine the carrier rate (Winata et al., 1995). A 25% carrier rate for the missense mutation of MYO15 predicts that among random marriages between two hearing people from Bengkala, 1.6% of the children will be deaf. This was calculated by multiplying the probability of two hearing parents from Bengkala being carriers (0.25 $\times$ 0.25) by the probability of their child being homozygous for the DFNB3 mutation (0.25) or (0.25 $\times$ 0.25 $\times$ 0.25 = 0.0156). This means we estimate that approximately 1.6% of the children born to hearing parents in Bengkala who have no deaf relatives will be profoundly deaf at birth. The higher than predicted incidence of deafness in Bengkala (2.2%) is, in part, due to assortative marriages among the deaf villagers. As a point of comparison, in the United States, epidemiological studies indicate that about 1 in 1–2,000 children is born with a severe hearing impairment, and approximately 50% are estimated to have a genetic cause for their hearing impairment (Marazita et al., 1993; Morton, 1991).

To what extent do mutant alleles of DFNB3 contribute to profound deafness in various populations worldwide? The missense allele of MYO15 causing congenital hearing loss in Bengkala, Bali is, so far, a private mutation, but clearly other mutations of MYO15 contribute to deafness beyond Bali. Two unrelated families segregating congenital hearing loss from India have been found to be homozygous for two different mutations of MYO15 (Wang et al., 1998). Preliminary data suggest that mutations at the DFNB3 locus may account for about 5% of congenital profound deafness in a sample of 82 families from India and Pakistan segregating nonsyndromic recessive deafness. The contribution of MYO15 mutations to profound hereditary deafness in North America is unknown. There is a bias in the types of families with hearing loss that have been ascertained, as the probands are typically profoundly deaf. It will be interesting, although difficult, to identify families with mild hereditary hearing loss. It is tempting to speculate that there are "mild" mutant alleles of MYO15 that cause either mild congenital hearing loss or progressive hearing loss.

FUTURE STUDIES

The presence of inner and outer hair cells in the *shaker-2* mouse, albeit with abnormally short stereocilia, offers the hope that the deafness phenotype may be reversed by treating these cells directly as opposed to germ line therapy. If a functional copy of *Myo15* could be introduced into the hair cells, would the stereocilia be restored to their normal lengths? If so, would the mouse then gain the ability to hear? These possibilities are now under investigation, and this work may eventually lead to treatments for people with DFNB3-related hearing loss due to mutations of MYO15.

Acknowledgments: The hospitality, consent and participation in this project of the families from Bali and India are appreciated. This work was supported by the National Institute on Deafness and Other Communication Disorders (Z01 DC 00035-01, Z01 DC 00038-01, and R01 DC 01634)) to TBF, EW, and YR, respectively, and the National Institute of Child Health and Human Development (R01 HD30428) to SAC. FJP is supported by a University of Michigan Rackham Fellowship. Jim Asher is included here as an author with permission of his wife, Doris. Jim died in May 1996 just days before our second trip to Bengkala to collect more clinical data and blood samples. We dedicate this chapter to his memory.

REFERENCES

Adato, A., Weil, D., Kalinski, H., Pel-Or, Y., Ayadi, H., Petit, C., Korostishevsky, M., & Bonne-Tamir, B. (1997). Mutation profile of all 49 exons of the human myosin VIIA gene, and haplotype analysis, in Usher 1B families from diverse origins. *American Journal of Human Genetics, 61*(4), 813–821.

Aksentijevich, I., Pras, E., Gruberg, L., Shen, Y., Holman, K., Helling, S., Prosen, L., Sutherland, G. R., Richards, R. I., Ramsburg, M. et al. (1993). Refined mapping of the gene causing familial Mediterranean fever, by linkage and homozygosity studies. *American Journal of Human Genetics, 53*(2), 451–461.

Avraham, K. B., Hasson, T., Steel, K. P., Kingsley, D. M., Russell, L. B., Mooseker, M. S., Copeland, N. G., & Jenkins, N. A. (1995). The mouse Snell's waltzer deafness gene encodes an unconventional myosin required for structural integrity of inner ear hair cells. *Nature Genetics, 11*(4), 369–375.

Baker, J. P., & Titus, M. A. (1998). Myosins: Matching functions with motors. *Current Opinion in Cell Biology, 10*(1), 80–86.

Ben Hamida, C., Doerflinger, N., Belal, S., Linder, C., Reutenauer, L., Dib, C., Gyapay, G., Vignal, A., Le Paslier, D., Cohen, D. et al. (1993). Localization of Friedreich ataxia phenotype with selective vitamin E deficiency to chromosome 8q by homozygosity mapping. *Nature Genetics, 5*(2), 195–200.

Brobby, G. W., Muller-Myhsok, B., & Horstmann, R. D. (1998). Connexin 26 R143W mutation associated with recessive nonsyndromic sensorineural deafness in Africa. *New England Journal of Medicine, 338*(8), 548–550.

Chishti, A. H., Kim, A. C., Marfatia, S. M., Lutchman, M., Hanspal, M., Jindal, H., Liu, S. C., Low, P. S., Rouleau, G. A., Mohandas, N., Chasis, J. A., Conboy, J. G., Gascard, P., Takakuwa, Y., Huang, S. C., Benz, E. J., Jr., Bretscher, A., Fehon, R. G., Gusella, J. F., Ramesh, V., Solomon, F., Marchesi, V. T., Tsukita, S., Hoover, K. B. et al. (1998). The FERM domain: A unique module involved in the linkage of cytoplasmic proteins to the membrane. *Trends in Biochemical Sciences, 23*(8), 281–282.

Cook, S. A., & Davisson, M. T. (1993). Re-mutation to shaker-2 (sh2). *Mouse Genome, 91,* 312.

Cope, M. J. T., Whisstock, J., Rayment, I., & Kendrick-Jones, J. (1996). Conservation within the myosin motor domain: Implications for structure and function. *Structure, 4*(8), 969–987.

Dobrovolskaia-Zavasdkaia, N. (1928). L'irradiation des testicules et l'heredite chez la souris. *Archives of Biology, 38,* 457–501.

Friedman, T. B., Liang, Y., Weber, J. L., Hinnant, J. T., Barber, T. D., Winata, S., Arhya, I. N., & Asher, J. H., Jr. (1995). A gene for congenital, recessive deafness DFNB3 maps to the pericentromeric region of chromosome 17. *Nature Genetics, 9*(1), 86–91.

Groce, N. E. (1985). *Everyone here spoke sign language: Hereditary deafness on Martha's Vineyard.* Cambridge, MA: Harvard University Press.

Kruglyak, L., Daly, M. J., & Lander, E. S. (1995). Rapid multipoint linkage analysis of recessive traits in nuclear families, including homozygosity mapping. *American Journal of Human Genetics, 56*(2), 519–527.

Lander, E. S., & Botstein, D. (1987). Homozygosity mapping: A way to map human recessive traits with the DNA of inbred children. *Science, 236*(4808), 1567–1570.

Liang, Y., Wang, A., Belyantseva I. A., Anderson, D. W. , Probst, F. J., Barber, T. D., Miller, W., Touchman, J. W., Long, J., Sullivan, S. L., Sellers, J. R., Camper, S. A., Lloyd, R. V., Kachar, B., Friedman, T. B., & Fridell, R. A. (1999). Characterization of the human and mouse unconventional myosin XV genes responsible for hereditary deafness *DFNB3* and shaker 2. *Genomics* 61, 243–258.

Liang, Y., Wang, A., Probst, F. J., Arhya, I. N., Barber, T. D., Chen, K. S., Deshmukh, D., Dolan, D. F., Hinnant, J. T., Carter, L. E., Jain, P. K., Lalwani, A. K., Li, X. C., Lupski, J. R., Moeljopawiro, S., Morell, R., Negrini, C., Wilcox, E. R., Winata, S., Camper, S. A., & Friedman, T. B. (1998). Genetic mapping refines DFNB3 to 17p11.2, suggests multiple alleles of *DFNB3*, and supports homology to the mouse model shaker-2. *American Journal of Human Genetics, 62*(4), 904–915.

Liu, X. Z., Walsh, J., Mburu, P., Kendrick-Jones, J., Cope, M. J., Steel, K. P., & Brown, S. D. (1997). Mutations in the myosin VIIA gene cause non-syndromic recessive deafness. *Nature Genetics, 16*(2), 188–190.

Marazita, M. L., Ploughman, L. M., Rawlings, B., Remington, E., Arnos, K. S., & Nance, W. E. (1993). Genetic epidemiological studies of early-onset deafness in the U.S. school-age population. *American Journal of Medical Genetics, 46*(5), 486–491.

Mburu, P., Liu, X. Z., Walsh, J., Saw, D., Jr., Cope, M. J., Gibson, F., Kendrick-Jones, J., Steel, K. P., & Brown, S. D. (1997). Mutation analysis of the mouse myosin VIIA deafness gene. *Genes and Function, 1*(3), 191–203.

Mermall, V., Post, P. L., & Mooseker, M. S. (1998). Unconventional myosins in cell movement, membrane traffic, and signal transduction. *Science, 279*(5350), 527–533.

Morton, N. E. (1991). Genetic epidemiology of hearing impairment. *Annals of the New York Academy of Sciences, 630,* 16–31.

Pollak, M. R., Chou, Y. H., Cerda, J. J., Steinmann, B., La Du, B. N., Seidman, J. G., & Seidman, C. E. (1993). Homozygosity mapping of the gene for alkaptonuria to chromosome 3q2. *Nature Genetics, 5*(2), 201–204.

Probst, F. J., Fridell, R. A., Raphael, Y., Saunders, T. L., Wang, A., Liang, Y., Morell, R. J., Touchman, J. W., Lyons, R. H., Noben-Trauth, K., Friedman, T. B., & Camper, S. A. (1998). Correction of deafness in shaker-2 mice by an unconventional myosin in a BAC transgene. *Science, 280*(5368), 1444–1447.

Schenker, T., Lach, C., Kessler, B., Calderara, S., & Trueb, B. (1994). A novel GTP-binding protein which is selectively repressed in SV40 transformed fibroblasts. *Journal of Biological Chemistry, 269*(41), 25447–25453.

Shuman, M. K. (1980). Culture and deafness in a Maya Indian village. *Psychiatry, 43*(4), 359–370.

Smith, C. A. B. (1953). The detection of linkage in human genetics. *Journal of the Royal Statistical Society, 15B,* 153–184.

Steel, K. P. (1995). Inherited hearing defects in mice. *Annual Review of Genetics, 29,* 675–701.

Titus, M. A. (1998). Coming to grips with a multitude of myosins. *Trends in Cell Biology, 8*(4), 171–172.

Wang, A., Liang, Y., Fridell, R. A., Probst, F. J., Wilcox, E. R., Touchman, J. W., Morton, C. C., Morell, R. J., Noben-Trauth, K., Camper, S. A., & Friedman, T. B. (1998). Association of unconventional myosin MYO15 mutations with human nonsyndromic deafness DFNB3. *Science, 280*(5368), 1447–1451.

Weil, D., Blanchard, S., Kaplan, J., Guilford, P., Gibson, F., Walsh, J., Mburu, P., Varela, A., Levilliers, J., Weston, M. D. et al. (1995). Defective myosin VIIA gene responsible for Usher syndrome type 1B. *Nature, 374*(6517), 60–61.

Winata, S., Arhya, I. N., Moeljopawiro, S., Hinnant, J. T., Liang, Y., Friedman, T. B., & Asher, J. H., Jr. (1995). Congenital non-syndromal autosomal recessive deafness in Bengkala, an isolated Balinese village. *Journal of Medical Genetics, 32*(5), 336–343.

3

Mouse Models and Progress in Human Deafness Research

Stacy Drury, Daryl Scott, Zhining Den,
Margaret M. DeAngelis, Mark A. Batzer,
Val Sheffield, Richard Smith,
Prescott L. Deininger, and Bronya J. B. Keats

For most of us mice are pesky creatures that invade our homes and startle us in the middle of the night. However, for many scientists mice provide powerful model systems for the study of mammalian physiology and genetics, which often enhance insight into human biology (Meisler, 1996). The study of the genetic causes of deafness is one research area that has benefitted substantially from the use of mouse models. This chapter discusses mouse models for human genetic deafness and focuses on our current studies of the *dn*, or *deafness*, mouse.

WHY THE MOUSE?

The similarities that make the mouse an excellent model system for human genetic research are not evident at first glance. However, closer examination reveals that the physiologic structures, including the cochlea and vestibular system, are remarkably similar between human and mouse, both in the developmental process and the functional adult structures. The DNA sequence and the organization of the genome itself reveal that we are not nearly as different from the mouse, at the molecular level, as we may think. Most of our genes are quite similar in DNA sequence, with some sharing upwards of 99% identity to the mouse counterparts, or *orthologues*. Additionally, the order and relationship of individual genes to neighboring genes in the human and mouse genomes are conserved. If, for example, genes A and B are located next to one another on a human chromosome, they are likely to be located next to each other on a mouse chromosome. Several computer databases (e.g., http://www3.ncbi.nlm.nih.gov) now provide lists of the locations of conserved regions and the genes they contain, making the identification of these similar genes even simpler. The simultaneous search for new disease genes in the human and mouse genomes has dramatically increased the speed with which disease-causing genes are mapped, identified, and characterized.

MOUSE MODELS AND DEAFNESS

More than 25 mouse models of deafness have been described and the locations of the defective genes within the mouse genome have been determined (Steel, 1995). Several of these mouse models map to the orthologous regions of human deafness loci and a database that lists these mouse models and the relevant human deafness loci is available (Van Camp & Smith, 1999; http://dnalab-www.uia.ac.be/dnalab/hhh). Mouse models have proven indispensable in the identification of three nonsyndromic deafness genes, two of which have been discussed in the preceding chapters of this book, and mouse models promise to be equally useful for other deafness genes (Petit, 1996). They offer several advantages over attempts to identify genes using only the human genome. First, the large number of controlled matings that can be set up with mice allows the development of a detailed genetic map. Second, samples for tissue-specific gene analysis can be accessed much more easily in mice than humans. And finally the selective correction or selective inactivation of specific genes using *transgenic* technology permits an exploration of gene function previously unavailable. This powerful tool has elucidated genes involved in the development of the auditory system for which naturally occurring mutations do not yet exist.

The first human deafness gene identified with the aid of a mouse model was the gene MYO7A that encodes myosin VIIa. Mutations in the orthologous mouse gene were found in the *shaker-1* mouse, and subsequently mutations in MYO7A were detected in patients with Usher syndrome type 1B and with nonsyndromic forms of hearing impairment (DFNB2 and DFNA11). MYO7A was the first gene identified that is involved in auditory transduction (Gibson et al., 1995, Liu, Walsh, Mburu, 1997; Liu, Walsh, & Tamagawa, 1997; Weil et al., 1995, 1997). Mapping studies in the *shaker-1* mouse and in Usher syndrome type 1B families provided the locations of the defective genes and suggested they were probably orthologues. The more definitive mapping information available for the *shaker-1* mutation localized the gene to a much smaller critical region in the mouse genome than the human data allowed and thus led to the isolation of the myosin VIIa gene in the mouse first. The significant cytoskeletal abnormalities in the *shaker-1* mouse made this gene a likely candidate, and the identification of the mouse gene provided the critical candidate for the human gene.

Myosins are mechanoenzymes that bind to actin and hydrolyze ATP to produce force. They are involved in a wide range of functions including movement, cell process extension, cytoskeletal structure, phagocytosis, signal transduction, and muscle movement (Probst et al., 1998). The detection of mutations in the gene encoding myosin VIIa, an unconventional myosin, in the *shaker-1* mouse and patients with several types of hearing impairment supports the importance of myosin in hearing. Since the identification of myosin VIIa, two other unconventional myosins have been implicated in the development of the auditory system (Avraham et al., 1995; Probst et al., 1998).

The second human deafness gene identified with the aid of a mouse model was DFNA15 (Vahava et al., 1998). DFNA15 is an autosomal dominant, adolescent onset, nonsyndromic hearing loss condition. The mouse model, in this case, is the result of a *targeted gene knockout* of the transcription factor POU4F3. Homozygous knockouts are profoundly deaf (Erkman et al., 1996; Xiang et al., 1997). Analysis of a family with hearing-impaired members mapped DFNA15 to a large region on the long arm of chromosome 5, but the presence of POU4F3 in the orthologous region on mouse chromosome 18 made it a strong candidate. Although no clear function of POU4F3 has been determined, it belongs to a family of transcription factors with a POU homeodomain and a POU specific domain that are both involved in binding DNA (Steel, 1998). Analysis of the POU4F3 sequence in DFNA15 family members revealed an eight base pair deletion leading to a premature termination of the POU4F3 gene product and removing the homeodomain. This mutation probably alters the function of the gene product by preventing DNA binding, but how this alteration leads to hearing impairment has yet to be elucidated.

Perhaps the most powerful feature of a mouse model is the ability to correct a phenotype *in vivo* using *transgenic* technology. This technology led to the identification of the gene encoding myosin XV as the causative gene in both the *shaker-2* mouse and DFNB3 families (Probst et al., 1998; Wang et al., 1998). The *shaker-2* mouse is an x-ray induced mouse mutation on chromosome 11 associated with profound deafness and circling behavior indicative of vestibular dysfunction. It was likely that the two genes were orthologues because four different genes in the *shaker-2* critical region mapped to the same human region located on the short arm of chromosome 17, which contained DFNB3. Transfer of the *bacterial artificial chromosome (BAC) contig* spanning the *shaker-2* critical region revealed a single 140-kilobase BAC that segregated with the rescue of both the deafness and the vestibular phenotype. Sequence analysis of the entire BAC led to the concurrent identification of myosin 15 as the *shaker-2* and DFNB3 genes. As the *shaker-2* mice exhibit dysmorphic stereocilia that are shortened but normally arrayed and the presence of an abnormal actin bundle in the hair cells, it is hypothesized that myosin XV is involved in the maintenance and organization of the actin within the sensory hair cells (Probst et al., 1998). Taken together, these three examples highlight the effectiveness of mouse models in the detection of human disease genes.

Many additional mouse deafness models exist that are not yet associated with human deafness conditions, including some for which the causative gene has been identified (Avraham et al., 1995; Street, McKee-Johnson, Fonseca, Tempel, & Noben-Trauth, 1998). Using transgenic technology to "knockout" or inactivate specific genes, new mouse models of deafness have been created that identify yet more genes crucial for the function and/or the development of the auditory system, similar to the method used in the *pou4f3* model. Knockouts important for development include Math 1, a gene essential for the generation of the inner hair cells of the cochlea, and the winged helix transcription factor Fkh10, a transcriptional regulator necessary for the early development of both the cochlea and the vestibulum (Hulander, Wurst, Carlsson, & Enerback, 1998). Additional knockouts of genes important for the correct functioning of the auditory system include Slc12a2, a secretory Na/K/2Cl co-transporter protein involved in endolymph secretion, and ATP6B1, an H+ ATPase involved in active proton secretion required to maintain endolymph pH, as well as distal nephron acid secretion in the kidney (Delpire, England, Dull, & Thorne, 1999; Karet et al., 1999). These knockout mouse models identify genes involved in the auditory system and highlight the importance of the maintenance of ion concentrations for correct auditory function and the role of transcription factors in the development of the components of the auditory system. As the number of genes involved in hearing increases we will be able to construct an interacting gene model for the development of the auditory and vestibular systems.

The *Deafness, dn* Mouse

The *dn* mouse is a model for human deafness with no other anomalies and no vestibular malformations. The *dn* mouse arose naturally in the curly-tail (*ct*) stock (Deol & Kocher, 1958) and has sensorineural deafness. The deafness phenotype in the *dn* mouse is inherited in an autosomal recessive manner, and *dn/dn* homozygotes are never able to hear. These mice do not exhibit the Preyer startle reflex or an auditory brainstem response (ABR) and are profoundly deaf from birth (Keats et al., 1995). In these mice one can see dramatic changes in the cochlear structure. There is marked degeneration of the organ of Corti, stria vascularis, and occasionally the saccular macula beginning at or before birth (Pujol, Shnerson, Lenoir, & Deol, 1983). By day 45 after birth, there is complete degeneration of the organ of Corti and no recognizable cell types remain. Interestingly, between day 45 and day 90, there is marked regeneration of the nonsensory cells, but only in the apical portion of the organ of Corti. One hypothesis for this local regeneration is the specific presence of GABA-nergic olivocochlear neurons only in the apical portion of the organ of Corti, which may promote regeneration (Bock & Steel, 1983; Pujol et al., 1983; Webster, 1985, 1992).

Electron microscopy studies show additional changes of the cochlea and inner ear of *dn/dn* homozygous mice. Transmission electron microscopic studies show shrunken and distorted inner and outer hair cells with vacuoles present in the cytoplasm. Scanning electron microscopy also detects an irregular arrangement of stereocilia, loss of most stereocilia, and giant cilia formation, similar to studies in another deaf mouse, the *Snell's waltzer*. The gene that causes deafness in the *Snell's waltzer* mouse has been identified as myosin VI, but a human deafness condition associated with myosin VI has not yet been found (Avraham et al., 1995). Finally the number of neurons in the spiral ganglion of *dn* mice is only 23% of that seen in heterozygous and normal hearing mice (Webster, 1985). The dramatic changes in the hair cells and the presence of abnormal stereocilia provide structural explanations for the electrophysiologic findings in the *dn/dn* homozygotes.

The endocochlear potential is normal in *dn* mice, demonstrating that sound is able to travel from the outer ear to the tympanic membrane. However, they exhibit no cochlear microphonics, suggesting a primary cochlear defect. Additionally, *dn* mice have preserved central auditory function on direct stimulation of the cranial nerve VIII, the vestibular-cochlear nerve, which is responsible for the transmission of sound to the brain (Bock, Franks, & Steel, 1982). Together these findings point to a fundamental defect in the functioning of the cochlear hair cells (Bock & Steel, 1983).

Interestingly although an occasional *dn/dn* mouse has been found with mild vestibular abnormalities, none exhibit the circling behavior characteristic of vestibular dysfunction seen in all other mouse deaf mutants (Bock & Steel, 1983; Brown & Steel, 1994). As the vestibular and the cochlear structures arise from the same embryological structures it is not surprising that deafness is often associated with balance problems. The lack of a vestibular problem in the *dn* mouse suggests that the gene causing deafness is likely to be involved either in the differentiation of the hair cells or the maintenance and functioning of the hair cells.

The Physical Mapping of the *dn* Region

Keats et al. (1995) localized the *dn* gene to the region containing markers *D19Mit14*, *D19Mit96*, *D19Mit111*, *D19Mit60*, and *D19Mit14* on mouse chromosome 19 and hypothesized the presence of a chromosomal *inversion* that disrupted the *dn* gene and led to the deafness phenotype. With this hypothesis in mind we began the construction of a physical map of this region to help us identify the structural changes on the *dn* chromosome as well as look for candidate genes that map to this region of the genome. The recombination data indicated that one of the breakpoints of the inversion is located between the genetic markers *D19Mit14* and *D19Mit96* (Vinas et al., 1998), and we therefore constructed a physical *contig* of this region.

Screening of the Whitehead mouse *yeast artificial chromosome* (YAC) library with markers from across the region identified a 460-kilobase YAC (91C10) that was positive for both *D19Mit14* and *D19Mit96*. This result demonstrates that *D19Mit14* and *D19Mit96* are probably within an interval of less than 460 kilobases. To further define the interval we used the polymerase chain reaction (PCR) to isolate clones from a total genomic mouse BAC library commercially available from Research Genetics, which contained the five markers *D19Mit14, D19Mit96, D19Mit111, D19Mit60,* and *D19Mit41*. Using PCR we determined which BACs overlapped with each other and were able to complete the contig (Figure 3–1).

The construction of this contig gave us the tools to further narrow the region of the breakpoint using *fluorescent in situ hybridization (FISH)*. This technique demonstrated that BAC 124J3 hybridized to two different loca-

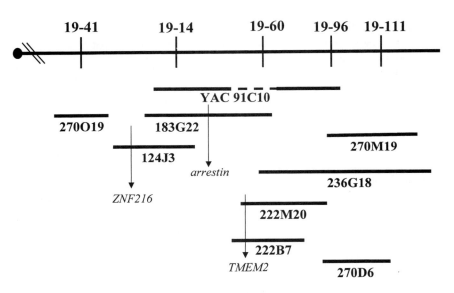

Figure 3–1. Physical map of the mouse chromosome 19 region that is likely to contain the *dn* gene. One YAC and 8 BACs that span this region are shown with their approximate locations below the entire chromosome. Specific genes that have been identified are in italics and are shown with line through the BACs on which they are known to be present.

tions on the *dn* chromosome 19, a result that is consistent with an inversion breakpoint being present on this BAC (Figure 3–2). Pursuing our hypothesis that the inversion disrupted the *dn* gene we have now focused our gene search on this BAC.

Candidate Genes in the *dn* Region and the Homology to DFNB7/11

The region of mouse chromosome 19 containing the *dn* gene is orthologous to a region of human chromosome 9 that contains the autosomal recessive nonsyndromic hearing impairment genes DFNB7 and DFNB11

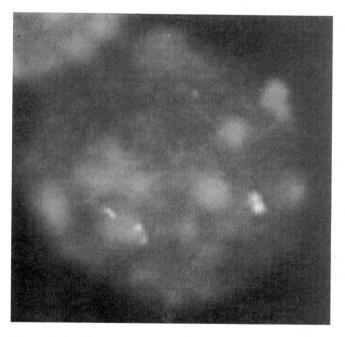

Figure 3–2. Fluorescent in situ hybridization (FISH) experiment of a cell from a *dn/dn* homozygous mouse using BAC 124J3 in blue and another BAC in a different chromosomal region in red as probes. There are four distinct blue signals but only two red signals, indicating that BAC124J3 is hybridizing to two distinct locations on each of the homologous chromosomes, while the other BAC is only hybridizing to a single location on both homologous chromosomes. This pattern of hybridization strongly supports the existence of an inversion.

(Jain et al., 1995; Scott et al., 1996). As it is likely that the mouse and human genes are orthologues, we began analyzing genes that are expressed in the cochlea and are located in the *dn* and the DFNB7/11 critical regions.

As the human EST mapping project has progressed faster than the mouse-mapping project and there exists a well-established human cochlear cDNA library, we were able to identify several human cDNAs that mapped to the DFNB7/11 region. Two of these cDNAs (ZNF216 and TMEM2) were shown to be new cochlear-expressed genes (Scott et al., 1998, 1999). ZNF216 shares homology with a gene that is involved in the development of the vessel endothelium from precursor cells and also with several genes that contain putative zinc finger domains. These domains are often found in DNA binding proteins. The function of TMEM2 is unknown but it contains at least one putative transmembrane domain. Sequence analysis using the NCBI Blast database (http://www.ncbi.nlm.nih.gov) identified the homologous mouse ESTs. Using both the mouse and the human EST sequences we were able to confirm the map location of both genes within the respective critical regions. Through direct sequence analysis of affected DFNB7/11 individuals we were able to exclude both TMEM2 and ZNF216 from causing deafness in these patients. In the mouse, we compared RNA expression in the brain of the *dn* mouse with that in the wild type (*ct*) mouse. Through *Northern* and *rtPCR* analysis we determined that there was no alteration in amount, size, or sequence of the RNA between the two mouse strains. Given these findings it is unlikely that either of these two genes are responsible for the deafness phenotype. However as these genes are both expressed in the cochlea, as well as a variety of other tissues, they may still play a role in hearing.

The extensive amount of DNA sequence and gene information available over the internet has dramatically enhanced the process of candidate gene analysis and more ESTs and cDNAs are being discovered and mapped every day. As well as ZNF216 and TMEM2 we have also eliminated *arrestin* as the defective gene. The protein encoded by this gene is thought to have an inhibitory role in the activated phototransduction cascade by interacting with either rhodopsin or a light-dependent cGMP phosphodiesterase. We are continuing to study other genes that map to the *dn* and the DFNB7/11 critical regions in order to identify the causative gene.

THE FUTURE AND TRANSGENIC MICE

The identification of genes that lead to diseases is an important area of research, but it is only the beginning of the process of understanding the defect and finding a therapy or cure for the disease. Once a gene has been identified at the sequence level the difficult process of dissecting the function of the protein encoded by this gene begins. One needs to examine not only the level of RNA and protein expression in different organs, but also the time in development at which they are expressed and the precise localization of the gene product both within the tissue and within the cell itself. Where exactly and at what times in the development of the cochlea is the *dn* gene expressed? Is expression limited to hair cells and the supporting cells in the cochlea or is there a wider expression distribution? What other genes interact with the *dn* gene and why is there degeneration of the cells after birth? These are just a few of the questions one can begin to answer once the gene is identified.

Perhaps the greatest advantage of using mouse models for research is the ability to put genes back into animals and see if one can correct the phenotype. Transgenic technology has rapidly advanced in the last 10 to 15 years. We have the ability now to not only put genes in and turn them off, but also to manipulate their expression at specific developmental time points and in specific tissues (Camper, 1987; Hogan, Beddington, Costantini, & Lacy, 1994).

We recently created transgenic mice containing BAC 124J3. By breeding these mice to *dn/dn* homozygotes we hope to cross the transgene onto the deaf mouse line and thereby correct the deafness phenotype. This technique has already proven successful in the *shaker-2* mouse and was instrumental in the identification of that gene (Probst et al., 1998). The existence of a transgenic model will greatly facilitate studies of the function of the *dn* gene as well as contribute to our understanding of the auditory system.

The search for deafness genes is far from over and it seems that there are more deafness loci than ever with new genes continually being identified. With the identification of genes causing deafness, research to determine their interactions with each other and the role that each plays in the auditory system is under way. Each gene is a small piece of the puzzle that will eventually give us a clear picture of how the intricate and delicate auditory and vestibular systems function and develop, and how a defect in a particular gene can lead to malfunctions in that process. It is only through a clear understanding of the molecular basis of deafness that we can design effective therapies and cures for this, the most common sensory deficit.

GLOSSARY

Bacterial artificial chromosome: Similar to the yeast artificial chromosome but containing a smaller amount of genomic DNA and replicating in bacteria instead of yeast.

cDNA: RNA is reverse transcribed into a single strand of DNA using reverse transcriptase and then made double stranded using the polymerase chain reaction. This double-stranded DNA represents the sequence of the gene without the introns.

contig: Overlapping pieces of genomic DNA contained in smaller vectors that are easy to manipulate to produce large amounts of a specific fragment of DNA.

EST: Expressed sequence tag. This is a small piece of RNA that is also made into double-stranded DNA and represents part of a gene. Several ESTs can be in a contig to give an entire cDNA sequence that represents the full length of the original RNA derived from a particular gene.

FISH: Fluorescent *in situ* hybridization. Using a small piece of DNA, a probe that is labeled with fluorescent antibodies, one hybridizes the probe to whole cells and a bright signal fluorescent dot is seen wherever the matching DNA sequence is found in the particular cell.

Inversion: A large fragment of a chromosome is inverted relative to the rest of the chromosome. For example, if there was a gene order: A B C D, and an inversion occurred between A and D, the new gene order would be: A C B D.

Northern: A method to detect changes in RNA size or amounts from a particular tissue or developmental time point of an animal. RNA is extracted from the tissue and electrophoresed in an agarose gel depending on the size of the RNA. Next the RNA is transferred and immobilized onto a nitrocellulose or nylon membrane. This membrane can then be hybridized with specific genes that are tagged with a radioactive marker so if they are present, a specific size and intensity of radioactive signal will be observed.

Orthologue: One of a set of homologous genes in different species.

rtPCR: reverse transcriptase PCR. A method used to amplify small quantities of RNA from a particular sample and convert the RNA to the more stable double-stranded DNA for further analysis. RNA is first extracted from a sample and then converted into single-stranded DNA using reverse transcriptase. Next the single-stranded DNA is amplified and converted to double-stranded DNA using the polymerase chain reaction, PCR.

Syntenic: The physical presence together on the same chromosome of two or more gene loci, whether or not they are close enough together for linkage to be determined.

Targeted gene knockout: The insertion of a gene or a piece of genomic DNA into a specific region of another animal's genome where it interrupts the endogenous DNA and stops the correct function of that gene.

Transgenic: The addition of a gene or a piece of genomic DNA directly into a fertilized egg of another species, which is then incorporated into a random place in that animal's genome and passed on to all the offspring of that animal.

Yeast artificial chromosome (YAC): A vector, similar to a normal yeast chromosome, that contains a large piece of genomic DNA from another species. The fragments range in size from 50 kilobase pairs to 1.5 megabase pairs of DNA. This vector can be replicated to produce large amounts of the specific fragment of DNA through the growing up of large amounts of yeast that contain the vector.

REFERENCES

Avraham, K. B., Hasson, T., Steel, K. P., Kingsley, D. M., Russell, L. B., Mooseker, M. S., Copeland, N. G., & Jenkins, N. A. (1995). The mouse *Snell's waltzer* deafness gene encodes an unconventional myosin required for structural integrity of inner ear hair cells. *Nature Genetics, 11,* 369–375.

Bock, G. R., Franks, M. P., & Steel, K. P. (1982). Presence of central auditory function in the *dn* mouse. *Brain Research, 23,* 608–612.

Bock, G. R., & Steel, K. P. (1983). Inner ear pathology in the *deafness* mutant mouse. *Acta Otolaryngologica, 96,* 39–47.

Brown, S. D. M., & Steel, K. P. (1994). Genetic deafness—progress with mouse models. *Human Molecular Genetics, 3,*1453–1456.

Camper, S. A. (1987). Research applications of transgenic mice. *Biotechniques, 5,* 638–650.

Delpire, E., England, R., Dull, C., & Thorne, T. (1999). Deafness and imbalance associated with the inactivation of the secretory Na-K-2Cl co-transporter. *Nature Genetics, 22,* 192–195.

Deol, M. S., & Kocher, W. (1958). A new gene for deafness in the mouse. *Heredity, 12,* 463–466.

Erkman, L., McEvilly, R. J., Luo, L., Ryan, A. K., Hooshmand, F., O'Connell, S. M., Keithley, E. M., Rapaport, D. H., Ryan, A. F., & Rosenfeld, M. G. (1996). Role of transcription factors Brn-3.1 and Brn-3.2 in auditory and visual system development. *Nature, 381,* 603–606.

Gibson, F., Walsh, J., Mburu, P., Varela, A., Brown, K. A., Antonio, M., Beisel, K. W., Steel, K. P., & Brown, S. D. M. (1995). A type VII myosin encoded by the mouse deafness gene Shaker-1. *Nature, 374,* 62–64.

Hogan, B., Beddington, R., Costantini, F., & Lacy, E. (1994). *Manipulating the mouse embryo.* New York: Cold Spring Harbor Laboratory Press.

Hulander, M., Wurst, W., Carlsson, P., & EnerBack, S. (1998). The winged helix transcription factor Fkh10 is required for normal development of the inner ear. *Nature Genetics, 20,* 374–376.

Jain, P. K., Fukushima, K., Deshmukh, D., Arabandi, R., Thomas, E., Kumar, S., Lalwani, A. K., Ploplis, B., Skarka, H., Srisailapathy, C. R. S., Wayne, S., Zbar, R. I. S., Verma, I. C., Smith, R. J. H., & Wilcox, E. R. (1995). A human recessive neurosensory nonsyndromic hearing impairment locus is a potential homologue of the murine deafness (dn) locus. *Human Molecular Genetics, 4,* 391–394.

Karet, F. E., Finberg, K. E., Nelson, R. D., Nayir, A., Mocan, H., Sanjad, S. A., Rodriguez-Soriano, J., Santos, F., Cremers, C. W., DiPietro, A., Hoffbrand, B. I.,

Winiarski, J., Bakkaloglu, A., Ozen, S., Dusunsel, R., Goodyer, P., Hulton, S. A., Wu, D. K., Skvorak, A. B., Morton, C. C., Cunningham, M. J., Jha, V., & Lifton, R. P. (1999). Mutations in the gene encoding B1 subunit of H+-ATPase cause renal tubular acidosis with sensorineural deafness. *Nature Genetics, 21,* 84–90.

Keats, B. J. B., Nouri, N., Huang, J. M., Money, M., Webster, D. B., & Berlin, C. I. (1995). The deafness locus (dn) maps to mouse chromosome 19. *Mammalian Genome, 6,* 8–10.

Liu, X. Z., Walsh, J., Mburu, P., Kendrick-Jones, J., Cope, M. J. T. V., Steel, K. P., & Brown, S. D. M. (1997). Mutations in the myosin VIIA gene cause non-syndromic recessive deafness. *Nature Genetics, 16,* 188–190.

Liu, X. Z., Walsh, J., Tamagawa, Y., Kitamura, K., Nishizawa, M., Steel, K. P., & Brown, S. D. M. (1997). Autosomal dominant non-syndromic deafness (DFNA11) caused by a mutation in the myosin VIIA gene. *Nature Genetics, 17,* 268.

Meisler, M. H. (1996). The role of the laboratory mouse in the Human Genome Project. *American Journal of Human Genetics, 59,* 764–771.

Petit, C. (1996). Genes responsible for human hereditary deafness: Symphony of a thousand. *Nature Genetics, 14,* 385–391.

Probst, F. J., Fridell, R. A., Raphael, Y., Saunders, T. L., Wang, A., Liang, Y., Morell, R. J., Touchman, J. W., Lyons, R. H., Noben-Trauth, K., Friedman, T. B., & Camper, S. A. (1998). Correction of deafness in *shaker-2* mice by an unconventional myosin in a BAC transgene. *Science, 280,* 1444–1447.

Pujol, R., Shnerson, A., Lenoir, M., & Deol, M. S. (1983). Early degeneration of sensory and ganglion cells in the inner ear of mice with uncomplicated genetic deafness (dn): Preliminary observations. *Hearing Research, 12,* 57–63.

Scott, D. A., Carmi, R., Elbedour, K., Yosefsberg, S., Stone, E. M., & Sheffield, V. C. (1996). An autosomal recessive nonsyndromic hearing loss locus identified by DNA pooling using two inbred Bedouin kindreds. *American Journal of Human Genetics, 59,* 385–391.

Scott, D. A., Drury, S., Bishop, J., Swiderski, R. E., Carmi, R., Ramesh, A., Elbedour, K., Srisailapathy, C. R., Lovett, M., Keats, B. J., Smith, R. H., & Sheffiefld, V. C. (1999). Refining the DFNB7/11 deafness interval using intragenic polymorphisms in a novel cochlear expressed gene, TMEM2. *Submitted.*

Scott, D. A., Greinwald, J. H., Marietta, J. R., Drury, S. S., Swiderski, R. E., Vinas, A. M., DeAngelis, M. M., Carmi, R., Ramesh, A., Kraft, M. L., Elbedour, K., Skworak, A. B., Friedman, R. A., Srikumari Srisailapathy, C. R., Verhoeven, K., VanCamp, G., Lovett, M., Deininger, P. L., Batzer, M. A., Morton, C. C., Keats, B. J. B., Smith, R. J. H., & Sheffield, V. (1998). Identification and mutation analysis of a cochlear-expressed, zinc finger protein gene at the DFNB7/11 and dn hearing-loss-loci on human chromosome 9q and mouse chromosome 19. *Gene, 215,* 461–469.

Steel, K. (1995). Inherited hearing defects in mice. *Annual Review of Genomics, 29,* 675–701.

Steel, K. P. (1998). Progress in progressive hearing loss. *Science, 279,* 1870–1871.

Street, V. A., McKee-Johnson, J. W., Fonseca, R. C., Tempel, B. L., & Noben-Trauth, K. (1998). Mutations in a plasma membrane Ca2+-ATPase gene cause deafness in deafwaddler mice. *Nature Genetics, 19,* 390–394.

Vahava, O., Morell, R., Lynch, E. D., Weiss, S., Kagan, M. E., Ahituv, N., Morrow, J. E., Lee, M. K., Skvorak, A. B., Morton, C. C., Blumenfeld, A., Frydman, M.,

Friedman, T. B., King, M., & Avraham, K. B. (1998). Mutation in transcription factor POU4F3 associated with inherited progressive hearing loss in humans. *Science, 279,* 1950–1954.

Van Camp, G., & Smith, R. J. H. (1999). Hereditary Hearing Loss Homepage. Available: World Wide Web URL: http://dnalab-www.uia.ac.be/dnalab/hhh

Vinas, A. M., Drury, S. S., DeAngelis, M. M., Den, Z., Huang, J. M., Berlin, C. I., Hunt, J. D., Batzer, M. A., Deininger, P. L., & Keats, B. J. B. (1998). The mouse deafness locus (dn) is associated with an inversion on chromosome 19. *Biochimica and Biophysica Acta, 1407,* 257–262.

Wang, A., Liang, Y., Fridell, R. A., Probst, F. J., Wilcox, E. R., Touchman, J. W., Morton, C. C., Morell, R. J., Noben-Trauth, K., Camper, S. A., & Friedman, T. B. (1998). Association of unconventional moysin MYO15 mutations with human nonsyndromic deafness DFNB3. *Science, 280,* 1447–1450.

Webster, D. B. (1985). The spiral ganglion and cochlear nuclei of *deafness* mice. *Hearing Research, 18,* 19–27.

Webster, D. B. (1992). Degeneration followed by partial regeneration of the organ of Corti in deafness (*dn/dn*) mice. *Experimental Neurology, 115,* 27–31.

Weil, D., Blanchard, S., Kaplan, J., Guilford, P., Gibson, F., Walsh, J., Mburu, P., Varela, A., Levilliers, J., Weston, M. D., Kelley, P. M., Kimberling, W. J., Wagenaar, M., Levi-Acobas, F., Larget-Piet, D., Munnich, A., Steel, K. P., Brown, S. D. M., & Petit. C. (1995). Defective myosin VIIA gene responsible for Usher syndrome type 1B. *Nature, 374,* 60–61.

Weil, D., Kussel, P., Blanchard, S., Levy, G., Levi-Acobas, F., Drira, M., Ayadi, H., & Petit, C. (1997). The autosomal recessive isolated deafness, DFNB2, and the Usher 1B syndrome are allelic defects of the myosin-VIIA gene. *Nature Genetics, 16,* 191–193.

Xiang, M., Gan, L., Li, D., Chen, Z. Y., Zhou, L., O'Malley, B. W., Klein, W., & Nathans, J. (1997). Essential role of POU-domain factor Brn-3c in auditory and vestibular hair cell development. *Proceedings of the National Academy of Science, 94,* 9445–9450.

Physical Maps as Molecular
Tools to Identify Disease Genes

Margaret M. DeAngelis, Chadwick J. Donaldson,
Gregory M. Ditta, Lauren M. Buckley, John P. Doucet,
Zhining Den, Stacy Drury, Mary Z. Pelias,
Prescott L. Deininger, Bronya J. B. Keats,
and Mark A. Batzer

Physical and genetic maps of markers are essential tools for gene localization and identification using the strategy known as positional cloning (Collins, 1991). The goal of positional cloning is to find a disease gene by determining its physical location in the genome without any knowledge of the function of the gene. Initially, linkage analysis of family data localizes the disease gene to a chromosomal region and determines the flanking genetic markers. From this information a physical map of genomic clones containing the flanking markers and the putative disease gene is constructed. Candidate genes are identified from the overlapping genomic clones and then subjected to mutational analysis in affected patients. This chapter reviews work from our laboratories to identify one of the genes responsible for Usher syndrome.

USHER SYNDROME

The Usher syndromes are a group of autosomal recessive disorders characterized by congenital sensorineural hearing impairment and progressive retinitis pigmentosa usually resulting in blindness. Although relatively rare in the general population, estimated at 4.4 per 100,000 in the United States (Boughman, Vernon, & Shaver, 1983), Usher syndrome accounts for 3–6% of children born with profound hearing impairment and accounts for over 50% of the adult deaf-blind population (Smith et al., 1994).

Three types of Usher syndrome have been differentiated based on clinical variation with respect to severity of hearing loss and vestibular impairment (Smith et al., 1992). Usher syndrome type I, the most severe form, is distinguishable from Usher syndrome types II and III by a severe-to-profound deafness and an absence of vestibular function (Smith et al., 1994). Usher syndrome type II patients present with moderate-to-severe congenital hearing loss (Smith et al., 1994), whereas the hearing loss in Usher syndrome type III is progressive (Davenport & Omen, 1977). Patients with Usher syndrome types II and III have normal vestibular function. All patients with Usher syndrome develop retinitis pigmentosa but the rate of progression may be variable. Histopathological studies of temporal bones of Usher patients show extensive degeneration of the hair cells of the organ of Corti and also the spiral ganglion cells (Cremers & Dellerman, 1988; Shinkawa & Nadol, 1986).

The chromosomal locations of nine of the genetic loci responsible for the Usher syndromes have been previously reported; however, only two of the genes have been identified to date (Van Camp & Smith, 1999). In 1995, the gene responsible for Usher syndrome type IB on 11q was found to encode an unconventional or nonmuscle myosin gene (Weil et al., 1995). Recently, the gene responsible for Type IIA on 1q was found to encode a protein with extracellular matrix motifs (Eudy et al., 1998). Type I Usher syndrome occurs in populations throughout the world, including a small southwestern Louisiana population descended from French-speaking emigrants exiled from Acadia. Our studies focus on the 11p locus for type I Usher syndrome in families of Acadian ancestry.

THE ACADIANS

In the early 1600s French fisherman from the northern coastal regions of France (Brittany, Normandy) settled in the Canadian territory known as Acadia (now Nova Scotia and surrounding areas). At the time of their expulsion (known as "Le Grand Dérangement") in 1755 by the British, the Acadian population had grown from a few hundred to nearly 20,000. Over the 40 years following this expulsion, approximately 4000 Acadians made their way to Louisiana (Rushton, 1979). These displaced people settled along the banks of the Mississippi River between New Orleans and Baton Rouge and on the plains among the bayous of southwestern Louisiana, where they remained relatively isolated because of linguistic, religious, and cultural cohesiveness, as well as geographic isolation. These factors are believed to have contributed to the higher frequency of Usher syndrome type I in the Acadian population than in the general population.

LINKAGE ANALYSIS

The gene for the Acadian form of Usher syndrome (USH1C) was localized to the p15.1-p14 region of chromosome 11 (Smith et al., 1992) and shown by linkage analysis to lie between the genetic markers D11S861 and D11S899, a distance of approximately 2 million base pairs of DNA (Keats, Nouri, Pelias, Deininger, & Litt, 1994). Ayyagari et al. (1996) refined the USH1C region to D11S902 to D11S1888. All affected individuals of Acadian ancestry have shown linkage to this locus (USH1C), and they are homozygous for the same haplotype at closely linked genetic markers suggesting a single mutation in the Acadian population (Keats et al., 1992). Nouri, Risch, Pelias, Litt, and Keats (1994) estimated that the USH1C mutation arose in the Acadians approximately 15 generations ago.

The family data analyzed in this study were described by Keats et al. (1994). The 46 affected individuals have a confirmed diagnosis of Usher syndrome type I and are of Acadian ancestry. They belong to 27 nuclear families from which a total of 54 disease and 50 normal chromosomes were available for analysis. Ten new genetic markers (D11S1397, D11S902, D11S4096, D11S4160, D11S4099, D11S1890, D11S4138, D11S4130, D11S1888, D11S1310) from the Whitehead Institute/MIT Center for Genome Research integrated map (Dib et al., 1996; Hudson et al., 1995) that are in the vicinity of the USH1C locus were used to refine the critical region by haplotype analysis. The 54 disease chromosomes had identical haplotypes from D11S902 to D11S4099. However, two chromosomes had a different allele at D11S1397 and one chromosome had a different allele at D11S1890. These results are consistent with the USH1C locus lying between D11S1397 and D11S1890, a physical distance of less than 400 kb on chromosome 11 (DeAngelis et al., 1998). More recently, DNA samples from additional Acadian Usher patients have enabled us to refine the critical region to a 200 kb interval between D11S4160 and D11S1890.

LIBRARY SCREENING AND
CONTIG CONSTRUCTION

Bacterial artificial chromosomes (BACs) have a number of properties that make them highly desirable for physical mapping. BACs are capable of faithful propagation of DNA fragments >300 kb in size (Ashworth et al., 1995; Kim et al., 1996; Shizuya et al., 1992). The BAC libraries are well suited for closing gaps in yeast artificial chromosome (YAC) maps using sequence tagged sites (STSs) as anchors to provide high resolution templates for subsequent large scale DNA sequence analysis (Ashworth et al., 1995; Kim et al., 1996).

Individual clones were isolated from total human genomic BAC libraries commercially available from Research Genetics (Releases I, II, and III). This library contains approximately 221,000 independent clones (average human DNA insert size 130 kb) arranged in a microtiter format of 72 superpools representing ninefold redundancy of the human genome. The human BAC library was screened by polymerase chain reaction (PCR) amplification of 21 genetic markers (D11S1397, D11S902, D11S4096, D11S4160, D11S1981, D11S1059, D11S921, D11S228, D11S4099, D11S1890, D11S4138, D11S4130, D11S1888, D11S1310, and D11S2450, 18b1(R), 966e8(L), KCNC1, 239h11 (L), BIR, and MYOD1) using primer sets previously described (Ayyagari et al., 1996; Dib et al., 1996; Hudson et al., 1995; URL: http://gestec.swmed.edu/human.html) and commercially available or custom made [Research Genetics]. All PCR amplifications were performed on BAC DNA and subjected to electrophoresis on an agarose gel to identify clones that contained each genetic marker (DeAngelis et al., 1998). Primers for 17 microsatellite markers (D11S1397, D11S902, D11S4096, BIR, D11S4160, D11S1981, D11S1059, D11S921, D11S1228, D11S4099, D11S1890, 18b1 (R), 966e8(L), D11S4138, D11S4130, KCN1, D11S1888) successfully amplified PCR products. No clones were obtained using markers D11S1310, D11S2450, 239h11 (L), and MYOD1. A total of 76 BACs were isolated using the 17 STSs, and 60 of these BACs were used to construct the contig across the region containing the USH1C candidate region (DeAngelis et al., 1998).

The region from D11S1397 to D11S1888 is covered contiguously with a minimum of seven BAC clones that span approximately 600 kb (Figure 4–1). Our complete map (comprising 60 BACs) represents a tenfold average coverage of the D11S1397-D11S1888 USH1C candidate region (DeAngelis et al., 1998) and is concordant with most of the other genetic and physical maps of this area (Ayyagari et al., 1996; DeAngelis et al., 1998; URL: http://www-genome.wi.mit.edu). The physical map of the short arm of chromosome 11 is our molecular tool to search for candidate genes.

CANDIDATE GENE ANALYSIS

There are several well-established methods that are complementary in nature for identifying coding sequence in a genomic region. Two of these methods are exon trapping and large-scale DNA sequencing of whole clones. DNA sequences generated from either of these methods are subjected to computational analyses to either predict coding sequence or search for identity with previously reported coding sequences in publicly available DNA sequence databases via the internet. Reverse-transcription-

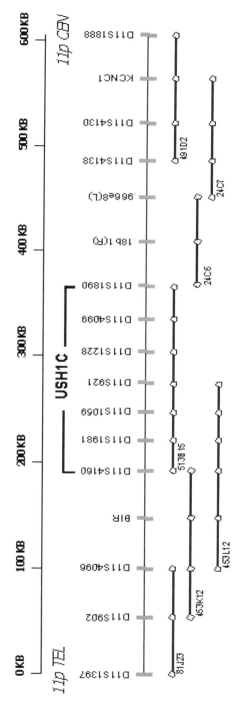

Figure 4–1. A BAC minimal tiling contig encompassing the USH1C critical region. The region depicted here from D11S1397 to D11S1888 is covered contiguously and minimally by seven BACs that span an approximate distance of 600 kb. The USH1C bracketed region indicates the area of the map that has been subjected to large-scale DNA sequencing. A scale of physical distance is denoted on the top line of the figure. Genetic markers are spaced along the genetic map in the second line of the figure according to the approximate physical distance between them. BAC clones are represented by horizontal lines beneath the genetic map of the region. Individual clones are identified by plate and well addresses directly beneath and to the left of the line segment and are scaled according to size. Open circles on a clone denote positive amplification for the genetic markers denoted by gray rectangles on the genetic map.

65

PCR (RT-PCR) is then used on human tissues and cell lines to demonstrate experimentally that the putative exons are actually protein coding. These methods are the first steps towards obtaining full-length cDNAs from candidate genes.

The first method we chose was exon trapping across our physical map of the USH1C candidate region. Exon trapping was performed on nine BACs spanning the USH1C critical region (DeAngelis et al., 1998). Putative exons were subjected to DNA sequence analysis (see Appendix). A basic local alignment search tool (BLAST) sequence comparison with confirmed exons revealed that only one shared a high degree of identity to a known gene, the human nuclear EF-hand acidic (NEFA) gene (Barnikol-Watanabe, 1994). To assess the possibility that expression of NEFA was associated with Acadian Usher syndrome, RT-PCR was performed on several human cell lines, including two lymphoblastoid cell lines derived from peripheral lymphocytes of patients with USH1C (lines GM10618 and GM10354 of the NIGMS Mutant Cell Repository), (DeAngelis et al., 1998).

We also performed comprehensive sequence analysis on cloned RT-PCR material to (1) confirm the identity of RT-PCR products as NEFA, (2) confirm the published sequence of NEFA cDNA, and (3) determine the nucleotide sequence of NEFA coding sequence from affected individuals. In comparing the full-length cDNA sequences that we generated, with the published NEFA cDNA sequence, no evidence for mutations in NEFA cDNAs from either affected patient was observed (DeAngelis et al., 1998). Therefore, we concluded that the NEFA gene is not likely to be responsible for Acadian Usher syndrome.

In parallel with exon trapping, we performed large-scale DNA sequencing on a BAC containing both flanking genetic markers D11S4160 and D11S1890. Computational analysis via BLAST and GRAIL, revealed 22 putative exons, 10 of which have statistically significant homology to known Expressed Sequence Tag (EST) clones in the NCBI and TIGR databases (http://www.tigr.org/tdb/hgi/hgi.html). Furthermore, the putative coding exons obtained by computational analysis have been analyzed experimentally for coding potential utilizing RT-PCR on several cell lines as well as human tissues from the brain and retina. This has not only enabled us to identify "true" coding exons but also to study the expression pattern of the various exons in order to prioritize them for further study. Of the 22 putative coding sequences predicted by computational analysis, RT-PCR analysis showed that 12 were true coding exons (Table 4–1). Furthermore 10 of the 12 exons have statistically significant matches to known expressed sequence tags (ESTs) in the NCBI (GenBank) and TIGR databases (Table 4-1). Unlike the NEFA gene that we localized to the USH1C critical region, the potential exons that we obtained from large-scale DNA sequencing did not share significant nucleotide identity with any previously

Table 4–1. Primer sequences (oligonucleotides) and NCBI/TIGR identification numbers for potential exons derived from single pass sequence data of one BAC in the USH1C candidate gene region.

Exon	GenBank I.D.	TIGR I.D.	Primer Sequence (5'–3')	Annealing Temp. (°C)	Size (bp)
Exon #1	N45082 W00864	THC150504	FOR: ATGAACAGCCAGTGGATTAGAA REV: TGATTGAGGTATAGGAAGGAAAAA	60°C	376
Exon #2	N49920	N49920	FOR: TACCACTCTACACAAAAGGCTACA REV: GGGTTCTGCACTATATGATTGAG	57°C	170
Exon #3	AA340458	EST45944	FOR: ACTGTCCTCCCTGCCTGGTG REV: TGGGGAACTTGGACGACTTT	60°C	224
Exon #4	N30385	N30385	FOR: TGGGGGCTCAAGGCATAG REV: AAAAGAAAGAAAGAGCGAATAG	57°C	182
Exon #5	AA708024	EST183098	FOR: ACCTGGCCTTATCCTTTCTTTTA REV: GTGGGATTATGGGATTTGTTTG	55°C	122
Exon #6	AA730310		FOR: GGAAACAGGTTAAGGTCACATAGT REV: AGAAGAGTAAACGGGACATCAAAT	57°C	188
Exon #7	AA680420 AA554066 T90277 R94708	THC94253 AA554066 AA001305	FOR: GAGTTTAATGATTGCAGGGTGACA REV: AATAAAACTACTGACTCTACTGGT	60°C	239
Exon #8	H78008 AA043051	THC292724	FOR: AGTGTGGATTGCTCTGAA REV: ATGATTATGTTATTGATGAAGG	52°C	737
Exon #9	T67639	T67639	FOR: TTGGGTGGAAAAGGAAACTG REV: GAAGAATTACCTACAAGAAACTG	55°C	141

(continued)

Table 4–1. *(continued)*

Exon	GenBank I.D.	TIGR I.D.	Primer Sequence (5'–3')	Annealing Temp. (°C)	Size (bp)
Exon #10	AA383629	EST97035	FOR: AAAAGCAGCAAGATCAAATA REV: TATTTTAGGGAGATATTGCTTC	53°C	154
Exon #11	GRAIL 2: 0.92	(Excellent)	FOR: GTCTTCCCTTCCACCATACATAA REV: GCCACAGCACCTACACT	58°C	231
Exon #12	GRAIL 2: 0.90	(Excellent)	FOR: TCGAAGCAAGACAGAAACCAAAGA REV: GGCAAAATATAAAAGAAGGGAAGG	60°C	145

Note: FOR denotes the forward or left primer and REV denotes the reverse or left primer. Annealing temperature is defined as the optimal temperature at which the primers hybridize to the target DNA sequence being amplified during a PCR reaction. Note that identification numbers are subject to change as the sequence data bases are updated on a daily basis. The computer search tool GRAIL is also subject to change based on updates of the analysis program.

sequenced genes contained in the NCBI or TIGR databases. In addition, we detected no changes in exon-specific RT-PCR or genomic PCR products from affected and unaffected individuals. Therefore we needed to obtain full-length cDNA clones in order to derive more sequence information for full-length mutation analysis in affected patients.

Presently, the exons we have identified are being used for (1) direct selection of a human fetal cochlear cDNA library and human adult retinal cDNA library, (2) Rapid amplification of cDNA ends (RACE) analysis of a human adult retinal cDNA library, and (3) PCR analysis of a human fetal brain library for obtaining full-length cDNA clones. Full-length cDNAs obtained by any of these methods will subsequently be used for mutational analysis in patients to precisely identify the gene responsible for USH1C. The identification of the USH1C gene will eventually provide important information for use in genetic counseling, as well as major advances in our understanding of hearing and vision.

Acknowledgments: This research was supported by a grant from the Foundation for Fighting Blindness to BJBK, MZP and MAB.

APPENDIX

There are two fundamental ways of finding genes in genomic sequence: (1) Homology-based methods search for similar sequences in current databases using the basic local alignment search tool (BLAST; URL: http://www.ncbi.nlm.nih.gov/; Altschul et al., 1990). (2) Feature recognition methods find potential protein coding regions using tools such as the Gene Recognition and Analysis Internet Link (GRAIL; URL: http://avalon.epm.ornl.gov/Grail-1.3/; Uberbacher & Mural, 1991). BLAST and GRAIL should be used together to effectively analyze sequence data. The BLAST programs used by the National Center for Biotechnology Information (NCBI) and The Institute for Genome Research (TIGR) work by first looking for similar segments between a query sequence and a database sequence, and then evaluating the significance of these matches.

GLOSSARY

Allele. One of the different forms of a gene at a given locus.
Bacterial artificial chromosome (BAC). A low copy number cloning vector propagated in bacteria that can carry DNA inserts 300 kilobase pairs or greater in length.

Complementary DNA (cDNA). DNA synthesized from an mRNA template, using reverse transcriptase.

DNA Clone. A segment of exogenous DNA inserted into a vector molecule, such as a phage or plasmid, and replicated to form many copies.

ESTs. "Expressed sequence tags" are partial sequences that are derived from cDNA libraries, with the objective of examining all expressed genes.

Exon. The transcribed regions of the gene that are present in mature mRNA and usually contain coding information.

Exon trapping. A method by which the protein coding portions of genomic DNA are expressed and cloned in vitro (Buckler et al., 1991).

GenBank. A comprehensive repository of sequence data and associated annotation built and distributed by the National Center for Biotechnology Information (NCBI) at the National Library of Medicine in Bethesda, Maryland.

Genotype. The alleles at specific genetic loci.

Haplotype. The combination of a group of alleles from two or more loci on the same chromosome, usually inherited as an unit.

Linkage. The association of alleles from closely spaced genes on the same chromosome from parent to offspring.

Polymerase chain reaction (PCR). A technique for amplifying segments of DNA. The method depends on the use of two oligonucleotide DNA primers and repeated cycles (30–40) of DNA replication using heat stable DNA polymerase.

RACE. "Rapid amplification of cDNA ends," a method by which full-length cDNA clones can be generated from knowledge of only a small portion of coding sequence.

Reverse transcription polymerase chain reaction (RT-PCR). A technique for amplifying mRNA for the purpose of obtaining cDNA. The method generally depends on the use of an oligo(dT) primer. This primer provides a 3' end that is used for extension by the enzyme reverse transcriptase.

STS. "Sequence-tagged site," a distinct location in the human genome, defined by two oligonucleotide primers that can be used in a PCR reaction to amplify this unique location in the genome. The sequence of the primers defines a marker at a particular site.

Yeast artificial chromosome (YAC). A cloning vector propagated in yeast, that can carry large DNA inserts up to one megabase in length.

REFERENCES

Altschul, S. F., Gish, W., Miller, W., Myers, E. W., & Lipman, D. (1990). Basic local alignment search tool. *Journal of Molecular Biology, 215*, 403–410.

Ashworth, L. K., Alegria-Hartman, M., Burgin, M., Devlin, L., Carrano A. V., & Batzer, M. A. (1995). Assembly of high-resolution bacterial artificial chromosome, P1-derived artificial chromosome and cosmid contigs. *Analytical Biochemistry, 224,* 564–571.

Ayyagari, R., Nestorowicz, A., Li, Y., Chandrasekharappa, S., Chinault, C., van Tuinen, P., Smith, R. J. H., Hejtmancik, J. F., & Permutt, M. A. (1996). Construction of a YAC contig encompassing the Usher syndrome type 1C and familial hyperinsulinism loci on chromosome 11p14–15.1. *Genome Research, 6,* 504–514.

Barnikol-Watanabe, S., Grob, N., Gotz, H., Henkel, T., Karabinos, A., Kratzin, H., Barnikol, H., & Hilschmann, N. (1994). Human protein NEFA, a novel DNA binding/EF-hand/leucine zipper protein: Molecular cloning and sequence analysis of the cDNA, isolation and characterization of the protein. *Biological Chemistry Hoppe-Seyler, 375,* 497–512.

Boughman, J. A., Vernon, M., & Shaver, K. A. (1983). Usher syndrome: Definition and estimate of prevalence from two high-risk populations. *Journal of Chronic Diseases, 36,* 595–603.

Buckler, A., Chang, D., Graw, S., Brook, J., Haber, D., Sharp, P., & Houseman, D. (1991). A strategy to isolate mammalian genes based on RNA splicing. *Proceedings of the National Academy of Sciences, USA, 88,* 4005–4009.

Collins, F. S. (1991). Of needles and haystacks: Finding human disease genes by positional cloning. *Clinical Genetics, 39,* 615–623.

Cremers, C. W. R. J., & Dellerman, W. J. W. (1988). Usher's syndrome temporal bone pathology. *International Journal of Pediatric Otorhinolaryngology, 16,* 23–30.

Davenport, S. L. H., & Omen, G. S. (1977). The heterogeneity of Usher syndrome [Publication 426, abstract 215, pp. 87–88]. Amsterdam: Excerpta Medica Foundation, International Congress Series.

DeAngelis, M. M., Doucet, J. P., Drury, S., Sherry, S. T., Robichaux, M. B., Den, Z., Pelias, M. Z., Ditta, G. M., Keats, B. J. B., Deininger, P. L. & Batzer, M. A. (1998). Assembly of a high-resolution map of the Acadian Usher syndrome region and localization of the nuclear EF-hand acidic gene. *Biochimica et Biophysica Acta, 1407,* 84–91.

Dib, C., Faur, S., Fizames, C., Samson, D., Drouot, N., Vignal, A., Millasseau, P., Marc, S., Hazan, J., Seboun, E., Lathrop, M., Gyapay, G., Morissette, J., & Weissenbach, J. (1996). A comprehensive genetic map of the human genome based on 5,264 microsatellites. Nature, 380, 2–154.

Eudy, J. D., Weston, M. D., Yao, S., Hoover, D. M., Rehm, H. L., Ma-Edmonds, M., Yan, D., Ahmad, I., Cheng, J. J., Ayuso, C., Cremers, C., Davenport, S., Moller, C., Talmadge, C. B., Beisel, K. W., Tamayo, M., Morton, C. C., Swaroop, A., Kimberling, W. J., & Sumegi, J. (1998). Mutation of a gene encoding a protein with extracellular matrix motifs in Usher syndrome type IIa. *Science, 280,* 1753–1757.

Hudson T. J., Stein, L. D., Gerety, S. S., Ma, J., Castle, A. B., Silva, J., Slonim, D. K., Baptista, R., Kruglyak, L., Xu, S.-H., Hu, X., Colbert, A. M. E., Rosenberg, C, Reeve-Daly, M. P., Rozen, S., Hui, L., Wu, X., Vestergard, C., Wilson, K. M., Bae, J. S., Maitra, S., Ganiatsas, S., Evans, C. A., DeAngelis, M. M., Ingalls, K. A., Nahf, R. W., Horton, L. T., Anderson, M. O., Collymore, A. J., Ye, W., Kouyoumjian, V., Zemsteva, I. S., Tam, J., Devine, R., Courtney, D. F., Renaud, M. T., Nguyen, M., O'Connor, T. J., Fizames, C., Faure, S., Gyapay, G., Dib, C., Morissette, J., Orlin, J. B., Birren, B. W., Goodman, N., Weissenbach, J., Hawkins, T. L.,

Foote, S., Page, D. C., & Lander, E. S. (1995). An STS-based map of the human genome. *Science, 270,* 1945–1954.

Keats, B. J. B., Nouri, N., Pelias, M. Z., Deininger, P. L., & Litt, M. (1994). Tightly linked flanking microsatellite markers for the Usher syndrome type 1 locus on the short arm of chromosome 11. *American Journal of Human Genetics, 54,* 681–686.

Kim, U.-J., Birren, B. W., Slepak, T., Mancino, V., Boysen, C., Kang, H.-L., Simon, M. I., & Shizuya, H. (1996). Construction and characterization of a human bacterial artificial chromosome library. *Genomics, 34,* 213–218.

Nouri, N., Risch, J., Pelias, M. Z., Litt, M., & Keats, B. J. B. (1994). Predicting the age of mutation for Usher syndrome type 1 in the Acadian population. *American Journal of Human Genetics, 55*(Suppl.), A160.

Rushton, W. F. (1979). *The Cajuns: From Acadia to Louisiana.* New York: Farrar Straus Giroux.

Shinkawa, H., & Nadol, J. B. (1986). Histopathology of the inner ear in Usher's syndrome as observed by light and electron microscopy. *Annals of Otology, Rhinology, and Laryngology, 95,* 313–318.

Shizuya, H., Birren B., Kim, U.-J., Mancino, V., Slepak, T., Tachiiri, Y., & Simon, M. (1992). Cloning and stable maintenance of 300-kilobase fragments of human DNA in *Escherichia coli* using an F-factor-based vector. *Proceedings of the National Academy of Sciences USA, 89,* 8794–8797.

Smith, R. J. H., Berlin, C. I., Hejtmancik, J. F., Keats, B. J. B., Kimberling, W. J., Lewis, R. A., Möller, C. G., Pelias, M. Z., & Tranebjaerg, L. (1994). Clinical diagnosis of the Usher syndromes. *American Journal of Medical Genetics, 50,* 32–38.

Smith, R. J. H., Lee, E. C., Kimberling, W. P., Daiger, S. P., Pelias, M. Z., Keats, B. J. B., Jay, M., Bird, A., Reardon, W., & Guest, M. (1992). Localization of two genes for Usher syndrome type 1 to chromosome 11. *Genomics, 14,* 995–1002.

Uberbacher, E. C., & Mural, R. J. (1991). Locating protein-coding regions in human DNA by multiple neural sensorineural network approach. *Proceedings of the National Academy of Sciences, USA, 88,* 11261–11265.

Van Camp, G., & Smith, R. J. H. (1999). Hereditary hearing loss homepage. http://dnalab-www.uia.ac.be/dnalab/hhh

Weil, D., Blanchard, S., Kaplan, J., Guilford, P., Gibson, F., Walsh, J., Mburu, P., Varela, A., Levilliers, J., Weston, M. D., Kelley, P. M., Kimberling, W. J., Wagenaar, M., Levi-Acobas, F., Larget-Piet, D., Munnich, A., Steel, K. P., Brown, S. D. M., & Petit, C. (1995). Defective myosin VIIA gene responsible for Usher syndrome type 1B. *Nature, 374,* 60–61.

5

Gene Therapy for the Treatment of Hearing Disorders

Julia L. Cook, Grace B. Athas,
Prescott L. Deininger

Gene therapy, or in vivo gene transfer, has tremendous potential to treat or cure human disease. The term gene therapy refers to the therapeutic delivery, not only of genes, but also of other nucleic acids (RNAs, derivatized DNAs and RNAs, oligonucleotides, etc.) that might modify gene expression. Gene therapy involves the delivery of nucleic acids into cells via transduction or transfection (viral vector- or nonviral vector-mediated nucleic acid delivery, respectively) to permit the production or repression of RNAs and/or proteins in either a continuous or regulated manner. Proteins generated from introduction of exogenous genes may function to compensate for abnormal or missing gene products characteristic of genetic diseases or to alleviate symptoms of nongenetic diseases through several different avenues. For example, overexpression of a gene product endogenous to a cell may augment the growth or tumor suppressor capacity of the cell. In addition, expression of foreign gene products can function to inhibit or augment endogenous gene expression, slow the rate of cell growth, inhibit viral replication, or induce cell death. Alternatively, it is possible to treat cells or tissues with "antisense" oligonucleotides or to introduce DNAs that express antisense RNAs, either class of which can anneal with specific complementary RNAs and decrease expression of the corresponding gene. These act either by inducing specific degradation or blocking translation of mRNAs (Gewirtz, Sokol, & Ratajczak, 1998; Kilpatrick & Phylactou, 1998; Laitinen & Yla-Herttuala, 1998; Morishita et al., 1998). Such treatments can be used to block aberrantly expressed genes, as might occur during viral infections or other disease states.

At the close of 1998, there existed 261 FDA/NIH submitted and/or approved human gene therapy protocols in the USA and 34 international

73

protocols (compiled in Human Gene Therapy, 1998). An examination of these studies shows that ~60% are for treatment of cancers, ~12% are for monogenic genetic diseases, and ~10% for treatment of infectious diseases. None of these protocols directly addresses hearing disorders. Some of the reasons for the current lack of clinical trials in this field are discussed at the end of the chapter.

Viral vectors are the most commonly used vehicles for in vivo gene delivery (see Friedmann, 1997; Karavanas, Marin, Salmons, Gunzberg, & Piechaczak, 1998; Robbins & Ghivizzani, 1998, for general reviews); the prototypes are the Moloney murine leukemia virus-based retroviral vectors (Gunzberg et al., 1998; Robbins & Ghivizzani, 1998). In NIH/FDA-approved protocols to date, retroviral vectors or retroviral vector producer cells have been most often proposed (>45% of protocols) as the mode of transduction. These vectors, however, are not readily taken up and expressed by the postmitotic sensory neuroepithelium of the inner ear and, therefore, will not be discussed further. We will instead focus on the viral vector systems that have shown the most promise in introducing genes to the inner ear. Adenoviral vectors (Ad vectors) are proposed in ~20% and pox viral vectors in 7% of the approved human protocols, to date the second and third most prevalent transduction mechanisms, respectively. Applications of naked DNAs and lipid-delivered DNAs account for ~20% of approved protocols (see Felgner, 1997; Gewirtz et al., 1998; Treco & Selden, 1995, for a general review of these methodologies). Most lipids designed for delivery of DNA are cationic. Lipids such as DOTMA (N-[1-(2,3-dioleyloxy)propyl]N,N,N-trimethylammonium choride) coat DNA to neutralize the negatively charged DNA backbone so that it is more readily internalized by cells (Treco & Selden, 1995).

In this chapter, we focus on systems that have already shown some promise for treatment of the inner ear.

ADENOVIRAL (AD) VECTORS

Adenoviruses, the etiologic agents of upper respiratory infections, possess a double-strand DNA genome of ~36 kb that encodes immediate-early proteins, (E1a and E1b), early proteins (E2–E4), and late proteins (Greber, Willetts, Webster, & Hellenius, 1993). These viruses attach to cells by their fiber coat protein through two identified and widely-distributed receptors (Bergelson et al., 1997; Hong, Karayan, Tournier, Curiel, & Boulanger, 1997; Tomko, Xu, & Philipson, 1997) and are internalized. Because the viral genome does not integrate into the cellular genome, cells can be "cured" of the viral infection, resulting in eventual loss of the transgene. Ad vectors have been derived from adenovirus by removal of genes whose packaging functions can be complemented *in trans* by recombinant cell lines expressing those genes. Removal of early genes, E1a and E1b (and sometimes E3), the products of which are required for replication, permits insertion of 7–8 kb of DNA into these vectors. Such vectors are referred to as first generation Ad vectors. In theory, they should be replication incompetent outside the recombinant cell lines that provide complementary functions. In practice, at high multiplicity of infection, cellular transactivators with compensatory E1-like activity may permit Ad vector replication (Imperiale, Kao, Feldman, Nevins, & Strickland, 1984). Accumulation of viral gene products may then initiate cytopathic effects and immune responses that may limit the duration of gene expression. These include activation of both CD8+ cytotoxic T lymphocytes and CD4+ T cells, the latter of which are required for development of a humoral immune response (Yang, Haecker, Su, & Wilson 1996). Thus, Ad gene therapy vectors permit only (predominantly) transient expression of the transgene, and treated individuals may develop an immune response which limits the effectiveness of successive treatments with adenoviral-based vectors.

Limitations of the first generation Ad vectors inspired the design of second (Engelhardt, Ye, Doranz, & Wilson, 1994; Zhou, O'Neal, Morral, & Beaudet, 1996), third (Brough, Lizonova, Hsu, Kulesa, & Kovesdi, 1996), and fourth (Ayres, Thomson, Merino, Balderes, & Figurski, 1993; Gu, Zou, & Rajewsky, 1993; Holt & May, 1993; Lieber, He, Kirillova, & Kay, 1996) generation, and gutless (Kochanek et al., 1996) Ad vectors in an effort to reduce cytotoxic effects and premature loss of transgene expression. These vectors were generated by deletion of progressively more viral genes, which were replaced *in trans*, in specific cell lines, to allow vector propagation. These vector systems accommodate recombinant inserts of anywhere from 10 kb to 28 kb, allowing expression of more, or larger, transgenes in a single vector. Some of these vectors have also permitted improved duration of gene expression and have been less immunogenic. Expression has been maintained in excess of 70 days with some of these vectors (Engelhardt et al., 1994).

Adenoviral vectors are being used with increasing frequency for several reasons. The first is the ubiquitous nature of the receptors; most mammalian cells, including those that are quiescent, can be targeted. This can be very important because, at any given time, only a small proportion of cells in the adult mammalian body are actively growing. Furthermore, some cell types, such as neurons, are terminally differentiated and no longer capable of proliferation. A second advantage is that Ad vectors can be purified to high titers (10^{11} to 10^{12} viable particles/ml for many derivatives), allowing infection of the majority of cells in a tissue. Potential disadvantages are the limited duration of transgene expression due to (a) cytopathic immune responses and (b) the fact that the vectors do not integrate into chromatin and may be lost during proliferation and cell turnover. The disadvantages may be minimized by the use of vectors deleted with respect to all viral genes; development and optimization of new vectors are ongoing.

Several studies have successfully utilized adenoviral vectors to transduce genes into the inner ear (Mondain et al., 1998; Raphael, Frisancho, & Roessler, 1996). These studies were all designed merely to demonstrate the degree to which various tissues in the inner ear can be infected with these viruses. The investigators employed a second generation Ad vector, Ad.RSV*ntlac*Z, which carries β-galactosidase as the transgene and expresses it using the Rous Sarcoma Virus (RSV) promoter. Because the promoter allows expression in a broad range of tissues, expression of the β-galactosidase gene acts as an indicator or reporter for cells that have been infected by the virus. Cells expressing β-galactosidase in their nuclei can be readily stained, and the number and types of cells expressing in a tissue can be visualized.

Raphael et al. (1996) injected the Ad vector into the cochlea of guinea pigs through the round window membrane (see Figure 5–1 for diagram). Seven days following the injection of approximately 10^8 adenoviral particles, the cochlea was harvested and stained with X-gal for β-galactosidase activity. Figure 5–2 shows the wide extent of staining obtained and demonstrates that a high percentage of cells throughout the cochlear spiral can be infected with this vector system.

ADENO-ASSOCIATED VIRUS

Adeno-associated virus (AAV) is a defective parvovirus that replicates in the presence of adenovirus or herpesvirus helpers. The host-range and tissue-specificity appear to be largely determined by the helper virus properties (Hermonat, Labow, Wright, Berns, & Muzyczka, 1984). The adeno-associated virus has a linear single-strand DNA genome of 4.7 kb. The DNA is flanked by 145 bp ITR (inverted terminal repeats), which are required for encapsidation of the virus. The wild-type genome preferentially integrates into human chromosome 19q13.3. The genome consists of rep (DNA replication), and lip and cap genes (encode proteins involved in capsid formation). Hermonat and Muzyczka (1984) first demonstrated that AAV could be used as a transducing vehicle. They ligated the neomycin phosphotransferase selectable marker under control of the SV40 promoter into an AAV plasmid genome deleted with respect to lip and cap genes. This plasmid replicated efficiently when transfected into adenovirus-infected cells. Packaging was accomplished by cotransfection of a plasmid (constructed to be too large to package efficiently) encoding required functions, although recombination between complementary regions in the two plasmids did result in limited wild-type genome generation. Significantly, despite the fact that wild-type AAV is silent (latent)

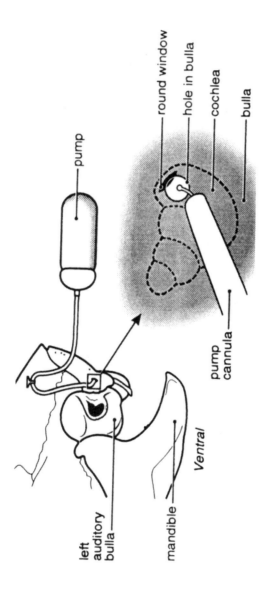

Figure 5–1. Introduction of vectors to the cochlea. This diagram shows the placement of an osmotic pump for introduction of reagents through a hole that can be drilled through the bony bulla structure for access to the cochlea. The osmotic pump allows injection of reagents over a prolonged period of time. Alternatively, vectors may be directly injected. (From "Osmotic Pump Implant for Chronic Infusion of Drugs into the Inner Ear," by J. N. Brown, J. M. Miller, R. A. Altschuler, and A. L. Nuttall, 1993. *Hearing Research, 70,* 167–172. Copyright 1993 Elsevier Science. Reprinted with permission.)

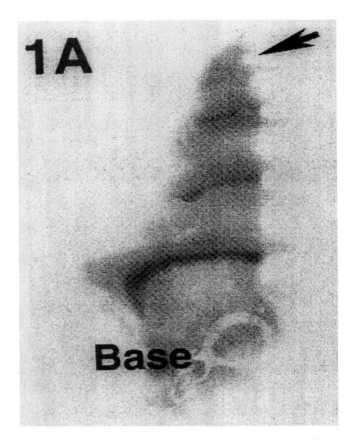

Figure 5–2. Transgene expression in the cochlea. This figure shows β-galactosidase expression in a guinea pig cochlea 7 days after injection of an Ad vector through the round window. These tissues were fixed and reacted with X-gal to display the distribution of β-galactosidase expression. Expression extends from the base to the tip of the cochlear spiral. (From "Adenoviral-Mediated Gene Transfer into Guinea Pig Cochlear Cells in Vivo," by Y. Raphael, J. C. Frisancho, and B. J. Roessler, 1996, *Neuroscience Letters, 207*, 137–141. Copyright 1996 by Neuroscience Letters. Reprinted with permission.)

when integrated, transgenes are efficiently expressed from the recombinant adeno-associated viral vector genomes. Other important features are that (a) titers of 10^{11} to 10^{12} infectious particles/ml can be obtained, (b) virtually any mammalian cell can be transfected, and (c) AAV are nonpathogenic and illicit a minimal immune response. The major limitation is that the packaging limit is ~5 kb.

Lalwani and colleagues have used recombinant AAV vectors for gene transfer into the guinea pig cochlea (Lalwani, Walsh, Reilly, Muzyczka, & Mhatre, 1996; Lalwani et al., 1997; Lalwani, Walsh, Carvalho, Muzyczka, & Mhatre, 1998; Lalwani, Walsh, Reilly, et al., 1998). Their first vector, pTR-MLPβ, encodes the reporter β-galactosidase and expresses the transgene under the control of the adenovirus 2 major late protein. This AAV vector was infused into the perilymphatic space of Hartley guinea pigs through a catheter placed in the basal turn of the cochlea (i.e., via a cochleostomy). An osmotic pump (Figure 5–1) was used to deliver 10^5 AAV particles in a volume of 100 µl over 8.3 days. β-galactosidase expression was detected by immunohistochemistry in the spiral limbus, spiral ligament, spiral ganglion cells, and the organ of Corti in the perfused cochlea, with a weaker and similar pattern of staining in the uninjected contralateral cochlea. The authors hypothesized that the appearance of staining on the contralateral side may be due to either a hematogenous spread, a spread through the bone marrow space of the temporal bone, or through cerebrospinal fluid that is in contact with the perilymphatic space through the cochlear aqueduct. The size of AAV may allow its spread in these compartments more readily than the larger Ad and HSV vectors. The viral spread of AAV to other tissues raises safety issues that must be addressed when considering this virus as a vehicle for gene transfer in the cochlea.

The same investigators have also used the green fluorescent protein (GFP) gene from *aequioria vitoria* as an alternative reporter gene in similar studies (Lalwani et al., 1997). The advantage of the GFP as a reporter is that it can be studied with fluorescent microscopy on living tissues and does not require any detection system that utilizes enzymatic assays or antibodies. In this study, utilizing the vector AAV-hrGFP(UF2), expression of the GFP was driven by the cytomegalovirus (CMV) immediate/early gene promoter and enhancer. Infusion of this vector system via cochleostomy resulted in intense fluorescence in the spiral ganglia, spiral ligament and limbus, Reissner's membrane, and organ of Corti.

HERPES SIMPLEX VIRUS (HSV) VECTORS

The HSV genome is a linear double-strand DNA of 152 kb encoding at least 75 gene products. HSV vectors have been used for gene transfer into explanted spiral ganglia and spiral ganglia in vivo (Geschwind et al., 1996; Staecker, Kopke, Malgrange, Lefebvre, & Van De Water, 1996). For these applications, defective HSV plasmids possessing an HSV origin of replication and a packaging signal (the plasmid is referred to as an amplicon) have been used (Geller & Breakefield, 1988; Geller & Freese, 1990). In the "defective HSV vector" system, the plasmid is packaged in a helper cell line, which typically supplies most of the required functions for replication (one gene, the IE3 gene, however, is supplied by a helper virus). The recombinant cells are transfected with plasmid and superinfected with a helper virus encoding IE3. IE3 is typically mutated (point mutation or deletion) such that its function is temperature sensitive. Growth occurs at the permissive temperature (typically 31° C), while no growth occurs at the nonpermissive temperature of 37° C (mammalian body temperature). In practice, some helper virus is generated during propagation of the HSV vector ex vivo, and during and after introduction in vivo. The ratio of helper virus to replication-incompetent HSV vector determines the cytotoxic effects and the experimental outcome. Major advantages of this system include (a) the ability of these vectors to readily infect postmitotic cells, (b) high levels of gene expression from multiple tandem copies of the transgene (typically 10–40, depending upon insert size) within the amplicon, and (c) an insert capacity of 15 kb or more.

Two studies have taken advantage of the neurotropism of the HSV vectors to infect cells in the spiral ganglion, both in vitro and in vivo (Geschwind et al., 1996; Staecker, Gabaizadeh, Federoff, & Van De Water, 1998). These laboratories created defective HSV vectors that possess the gene for brain-derived neurotrophic factor (BDNF). BDNF is important to the maturation and function of mammalian auditory neurons and plays an important role in innervation of the developing cochlea (Ernfors, Duan, ElShamy, & Canlon, 1996). BDNF has previously been shown to protect against the loss of auditory neurons when the inner ear is damaged (Staecker et al., 1996). One of these vectors also possessed the gene for β-galactosidase, so that the vector could express both BDNF for neural protection and a reporter gene for determining the type and proportion of infected cells. To test for biological activity, the constructs were incubated with growth factor-dependent cell lines, neuronal cells, and spiral ganglion explant cultures. Both vector constructs were capable of supporting cell survival and growth, and neurite extension. They were shown to infect both neuronal and nonneuronal cells, resulting in production of functional BDNF.

The BDNF-producing herpes vectors were then used in a mouse model in which the inner ear was subjected to an ototoxic neomycin treatment through a cochleostomy. The ototoxic treatment destroys the hair cells that normally produce neuroprotective factors and results in neuronal degeneration. Subsequently, the ear in these animals was infused with the herpes vector or saline. Four weeks after injection of these agents, strong expression of β-galactosidase was detected by immunohistochemistry, particularly in the spiral ganglion. This included about 50% of the neural cells, as well as non-neural cells in the spiral ganglion, endothelial cells, and the stria vascularis. Most importantly, numbers of auditory neurons were greatly enhanced in organs that received the BDNF-producing herpes vector. This study provides an exciting example of how gene therapy may successfully be used in a clinical situation.

NON-VIRAL GENE THERAPY

In a recent study, the cationic liposome, dimethyldioctadecylammonium bromide (DDAB), was employed to introduce the reporter gene, β-galactosidase, into the guinea pig cochlea (Wareing et al., 1999). Liposomes coat DNA molecules and assist their uptake into cells. Complexes were introduced to the cochea either by direct injection or infusion through a cochleostomy, and transgene expression was examined at 1, 3, 7, and 14 days. Immunoreactivity to polyclonal β-galactosidase antibodies was detected at 3, 7, and 14 days. Nearly all tissue types were positive for β-galactosidase expression, including the tissue surrounding the cochlear duct; the bony modiolus from base to apex; and spiral ligament, spiral limbus, and organ of Corti (including outer hair cells as well as supporting cells, Reissner's membrane, and auditory neurons within the spiral ganglion). The stria vascularis did not display β-galactosidase immunoreactivity. The intensity of β-galactosidase expression was greater at 7 days versus 14 days. Animals infused with liposomes devoid of the β-galactosidase plasmid, as well as saline-injected animals, displayed no immunoreactivity. In addition, animals that were given a direct slow injection (10 μl over 20 min) exhibited no inflammatory reaction as detected by T-cell immunoreactivity. Animals infused with β-galactosidase liposomes using the cochleostomy and mini-osmotic pump (100 μl over 8.3 days) showed fibrosis and an acute immune response localized at the site of the cochleostomy.

The presence of reporter gene in the contralateral ear was also assessed by PCR on DNA extracted from paraffin-embedded cochlear sections. The 450-bp β-galactosidase amplification product was detected in the ipsilateral (injected) cochlea at 1, 3, 7, and 14 days, but not in the contralateral cochlea. The absence of reporter gene in the contralateral cochlea may be due to the large size (260–560 nm in diameter) of liposome complexes which may prevent dissemination of the nature observed in studies (previously cited) with AAV (15–20 nm diameter).

Another nonviral approach that has been used to modify gene expression in the inner ear involves antisense oligonucleotides. These molecules are designed to pair with and degrade or inhibit translation of specific mRNA molecules. Thus, in theory, it is possible to down-regulate the expression of any specific gene with this approach. In practice, a number of nonspecific effects have been associated with many of these oligonucleotides (Flanagan, 1998), and developments to improve both the efficacy and specificity of this approach are ongoing. Unlike viral delivery systems, which can express genes for long periods of time, antisense oligonucleotides are generally fairly unstable and are only effective if continuously delivered. Thus, most studies have used an osmotic minipump delivery system. Antisense oligonucleotides have been effectively delivered to the inner ear to decrease expression of the GluR2 AMPA receptor (d'Aldin et al., 1998), FGF3 (Frenz & Liu, 1998), and NGF, BDNF and NT-3 (Frenz & Liu, 1998; Staecker et al., 1996). Although this approach has been used predominantly as a research tool to test the influence of these genes on the development and function of the inner ear, these examples demonstrate the potential to use such a delivery system in a therapeutic manner as well.

THE FUTURE OF GENE THERAPY FOR HEARING DISORDERS

A number of factors make gene therapy for hearing disorders very attractive. Several issues are also likely to limit the utility of gene therapy for hearing disorders. The biggest attraction is that the inner ear contains a fluid-filled space that accesses all of the relevant cell types for treatment. This allows efficient delivery of gene therapy vectors to a very high proportion of the cells in the inner ear, as demonstrated by all of the studies discussed above (see Figure 5–2). In addition, gene therapy vectors can be readily contained within this structure, minimizing the potential dangers of altering gene expression in other parts of the body with potentially adverse effects. Vector and delivery systems are available that will allow the efficient delivery of genes to a broad range of cell types in the inner ear. Although future improvements are likely, vector design does not seem to be a limiting factor at this point. Ultimately, vector refinements that lessen cytotoxic effects, or allow for increased length of expression or more highly regulated expression of the transgenes, will allow therapies for a broader range of disorders. However, the studies in which BDNF expression was found to protect against nerve damage in response to antibiotic treatments (Geschwind et al., 1996; Staecker et al., 1998) demonstrate that practical effects can be obtained with gene therapy in the inner ear.

One factor that will limit human gene therapy trials for inner ear defects for some time is that hearing disorders tend not to be life threatening. Most of the early gene therapy trials have been performed for life-threatening disorders because of the many uncertainties of applying novel technologies. It is critical that no side effect of the treatment be worse than the disease being treated. As investigators gain confidence in the safety of gene therapy, protocols will begin to appear for less serious disorders.

One of the biggest hurdles to overcome in gene therapy for hearing disorders is the complex and delicate nature of the hearing apparatus itself. This structure develops in the embryo through a series of very complex cellular interactions. Many hearing disorders involve genetic defects or traumas that alter the development of the inner ear. It is likely to be very difficult to find gene therapy approaches that can appropriately direct the complex development of these structures. It would be a challenge to direct gene therapy in a controlled enough manner to repair developmental defects in the embryo, even were there not tremendous difficulties and potential risks associated with gene delivery at early developmental stages. Thus, gene therapies to repair developmental difficulties or to regenerate complex hair cell structures are likely to be difficult or impossible in the near future.

Currently the types of gene therapies that seem promising are those that involve either genetic defects or traumas that result in degeneration of cochlear structures after they have developed. Introducing genes that protect the cochlea from degeneration is already possible for some forms of nerve degeneration, and it seems quite possible to effectively replace defective genes that can contribute to these later onset forms of deafness.

The beauty of gene delivery as a therapeutic option is that, with an appropriate understanding of the biology of the inner ear, we should have an incredible wealth of options to use in new therapies. The limitations are that we still know too little about the interacting factors that might prove useful when encoded by therapeutic transgenes, as well as the fine points of delivery and transgene expression optimization.

REFERENCES

Anonymous. (1998). Human gene marker/therapy clinical protocols. *Human Gene Therapy, 9*, 2805–2852.

Ayres, E. K., Thomson, V. J., Merino, G., Balderes, D., & Figurski, D. H. (1993). Precise deletions in large bacterial genomes by vector-mediated excision (VEX). The trfA gene of promiscuous plasmid RK2 is essential for replication in several gram-negative hosts. *Journal of Molecular Biology, 230*, 174–185.

Bergelson, J. M., Cunningham, J. A., Droguett, G., Kurt-Jones, E. A., Krithivas, A., Hong, J. S., Horwitz, M. S., Crowell, R. L., & Finberg, R. W. (1997). Isolation of a common receptor for Coxsackie B viruses and adenoviruses 2 and 5. *Science, 275*, 1320–1323.

Brough, D. E., Lizonova, A., Hsu, C., Kulesa, V. A., & Kovesdi, I. (1996). A gene transfer vector-cell line system for complete functional complementation of adenovirus early regions E1 and E4. *Journal of Virology, 70*, 6497–6501.

d'Aldin, C., Caicedo, A., Ruel, J., Renard, N., Pujol, R., & Puel, J. L. (1998). Antisense oligonucleotides to the GluR2 AMPA receptor subunit modify excitatory synaptic transmission in vivo. *Brain Research and Molecular Brain Research, 55*, 151–164.

Engelhardt, J. F., Ye, X., Doranz, B., & Wilson, J. M. (1994). Ablation of E2A in recombinant adenoviruses improves transgene persistence and decreases inflammatory response in mouse liver. *Proceedings of the National Academy of Science, USA, 91*, 6196–6200.

Ernfors, P., Duan, M. L., ElShamy, W. M., & Canlon, B. (1996). Protection of auditory neurons from aminoglycoside toxicity by neurotrophin-3. *Nature Medicine, 2*, 463–467.

Felgner, P. L. (1997). Nonviral strategies for gene therapy. *Scientific American, 276,* 102–106.

Flanagan, W. M. (1998). Antisense comes of age. *Cancer Metastasis Review, 17*(2), 169–176.

Frenz, D. A., & Liu, W. (1998). Role of FGF3 in otic capsule chondrogenesis in vitro: An antisense oligonucleotide approach. *Growth Factors, 15,* 173–182.

Friedmann, T. (1997). Overcoming the obstacles to gene therapy. *Scientific American, 276,* 96–101.

Geller, A. I., & Breakefield, X. O. (1988). A defective HSV-1 vector expresses *Escherichia* coli beta-galactosidase in cultured peripheral neurons. *Science, 241,* 1667–1669.

Geller, A. I., & Freese, A. (1990). Infection of cultured central nervous system neurons with a defective herpes simplex virus 1 vector results in stable expression of *Escherichia* coli betagalactosidase. *Proceedings of the National Academy of Science USA, 87,* 1149–1153.

Geschwind, M. D., Hartnick, C. J., Liu, W., Amat, J., Van De Water, T. R., & Federoff, H. J. (1996). Defective HSV-1 vector expressing BDNF in auditory ganglia elicits neurite outgrowth: Model for treatment of neuron loss following cochlear degeneration. *Human Gene Therapy, 7,* 173–182.

Gewirtz, A. M., Sokol, D. L., & Ratajczak, M. Z. (1998). Nucleic acid therapeutics: State of the art and future prospects. *Blood, 92,* 712–736.

Greber, U. F., Willetts, M., Webster, P., & Helenius, A. (1993). Stepwise dismantling of adenovirus 2 during entry into cells. *Cell, 75,* 477–486.

Gu, H., Zou, Y. R., & Rajewsky, K. (1993). Independent control of immunoglobulin switch recombination at individual switch regions evidenced through Cre-loxP-mediated gene targeting. *Cell, 73,* 1155–1164.

Gunzburg, W. H., Karle, P., Mrochen, S., Sparmann, G., Saller, R., Klein, D., Uckert, W., & Salmons, B. (1998). Regulated gene expression after retroviral vector-mediated delivery of cancer-relevant therapeutic genes. *Recent Results in Cancer Research, 144,* 116–126.

Hermonat, P. L., Labow, M. A., Wright, R., Berns, K. I., & Muzyczka, N. (1984). Genetics of adeno-associated virus: Isolation and preliminary characterization of adeno-associated virus type 2 mutants. *Journal of Virology, 51,* 329–339.

Hermonat, P. L., & Muzyczka, N. (1984). Use of adeno-associated virus as a mammalian DNA cloning vector: Transduction of neomycin resistance into mammalian tissue culture cells. *Proceedings of the National Academy of Science, USA, 81,* 6466–6470.

Holt, C. L., & May, G. S. (1993). A novel phage lambda replacement Cre-lox vector that has automatic subcloning capabilities. *Gene, 133,* 95–97.

Hong, S. S., Karayan, L., Tournier, J., Curiel, D. T., & Boulanger, P. A. (1997). Adenovirus type 5 fiber knob binds to MHC class I alpha2 domain at the surface of human epithelial and B lymphoblastoid cells. *EMBO Journal, 16,* 2294–2306.

Imperiale, M. J., Kao, H. T., Feldman, L. T., Nevins, J. R., & Strickland, S. (1984). Common control of the heat shock gene and early adenovirus genes: Evidence for a cellular E1A-like activity. *Molecular and Cell Biology, 4,* 867–874.

Karavanas, G., Marin, M., Salmons, B., Gunzburg, W. H., & Piechaczyk, M. (1998). Cell targeting by murine retroviral vectors. *Critical Reviews in Oncology and Hematology, 28,* 7–30.

Kilpatrick, M. W., & Phylactou, L. A. (1998). Towards an RNA-based therapy for Marfan syndrome. *Molecular Medicine Today, 4,* 376–381.

Kochanek, S., Clemens, P. R., Mitani, K., Chen, H. H., Chan, S., & Caskey, C. T. (1996). A new adenoviral vector: Replacement of all viral coding sequences with 28 kb of DNA independently expressing both full-length dystrophin and beta-galactosidase. *Proceedings of the National Academy of Science USA, 93,* 5731-5736.

Laitinen, M., & Yla-Herttuala, S. (1998). Vascular gene transfer for the treatment of restenosis and atherosclerosis. *Current Opinions in Lipidology, 9,* 465–469.

Lalwani, A. K., Han, J. J., Walsh, B. J., Zolotukhin, S., Muzyczka, N., & Mhatre, A. N. (1997). Green fluorescent protein as a reporter for gene transfer studies in the cochlea. *Hearing Research, 114,* 139–147.

Lalwani, A. K., Walsh, B. J., Carvalho, G. J., Muzyczka, N., & Mhatre, A. N. (1998). Expression of adeno-associated virus integrated transgene within the mammalian vestibular organs. *American Journal of Otology, 19,* 390-395.

Lalwani, A., Walsh, B., Reilly, P., Carvalho, G., Zolotukhin, S., Muzyczka, N., & Mhatre, A. (1998). Long-term in vivo cochlear transgene expression mediated by recombinant adeno-associated virus. *Gene Therapy, 5,* 277–281.

Lalwani, A. K., Walsh, B. J., Reilly, P. G., Muzyczka, N., & Mhatre, A. N. (1996). Development of in vivo gene therapy for hearing disorders: Introduction of adeno-associated virus into the cochlea of the guinea pig. *Gene Therapy, 3,* 588–592.

Lieber, A., He, C. Y., Kirillova, I., & Kay, M. A. (1996). Recombinant adenoviruses with large deletions generated by Cre-mediated excision exhibit different biological properties compared with first-generation vectors in vitro and in vivo. *Journal of Virology, 70,* 8944–8960.

Mondain, M., Restituito, S., Vincenti, V., Gardiner, Q., Uziel, A., Delabre, A., Mathieu, M., Bousquet, J., & Demoly, P. (1998). Adenovirus-mediated in vivo gene transfer in guinea pig middle ear mucosa. *Human Gene Therapy, 9,* 1217–1221.

Morishita, R., Nakagami, H., Taniyama, Y., Matsushita, H., Yamamoto, K., Tomita, N., Moriguchi, A., Matsumoto, K., Higaki, J., & Ogihara, T. (1998). Oligonucleotide-based gene therapy for cardiovascular disease. *Clinical Chemistry and Laboratory Medicine, 36,* 529–534.

Raphael, Y., Frisancho, J. C., & Roessler, B. J. (1996). Adenoviral-mediated gene transfer into guinea pig cochlear cells in vivo. *Neuroscience Letters, 207,* 137–141.

Robbins, P. D., & Ghivizzani, S. C. (1998). Viral vectors for gene therapy. *Pharmacology Therapy, 80,* 35–47.

Staecker, H., Gabaizadeh, R., Federoff, H., & Van De Water, T. R. (1998). Brain-derived neurotrophic factor gene therapy prevents spiral ganglion degeneration after hair cell loss. *Otolaryngology—Head and Neck Surgery, 119,* 7–13.

Staecker, H., Kopke, R., Malgrange, B., Lefebvre, P., & Van De Water, T. R. (1996). NT-3 and/or BDNF therapy prevents loss of auditory neurons following loss of hair cells. *Neuroreport, 7,* 889–894.

Staecker, H., Van De Water, T. R., Lefebvre, P. P., Liu, W., Moghadassi, M., Galinovic-Schwartz, V., Malgrange, B., & Moonen, G. (1996). NGF, BDNF and NT-3 play unique roles in the in vitro development and patterning of innervation of the mammalian inner ear. *Brain Research, Developmental Brain Research, 92,* 49–60.

Tomko, R. P., Xu, R., & Philipson, L. (1997). HCAR and MCAR: The human and mouse cellular receptors for subgroup C adenoviruses and group B coxsackieviruses. *Proceedings of the National Academy of Science, USA, 94,* 3352–3356.

Treco, D. A., & Selden, R. F. (1995). Non-viral gene therapy. *Molecular Medicine Today, 1*, 314–321.

Wareing, M., Mhatre, A. N., Pettis, R., Han, J. J., Haut, T., Pfister, M. H., Hong, K., Zheng, W. W., & Lalwani, A. K. (1999). Cationic liposome mediated transgene expression in the guinea pig cochlea. *Hearing Research, 128*, 61–69.

Yang, Y., Haecker, S. E., Su, Q., & Wilson, J. M. (1996). Immunology of gene therapy with adenoviral vectors in mouse skeletal muscle. *Human Molecular Genetics, 5*, 1703–1712.

Zhou, H., O'Neal, W., Morral, N., & Beaudet, A. L. (1996). Development of a complementing cell line and a system for construction of adenovirus vectors with E1 and E2a deleted. *Journal of Virology, 70*, 7030–7038.

Transmitters in the Cochlea: ATP as a Neuromodulator in the Organ of Corti

Richard P. Bobbin, Anthony P. Barnes, Chu Chen,
Prescott L. Deininger, Christopher S. LeBlanc,
and Margaret S. Parker

The functions of various chemicals in the cochlea are slowly being defined. For example, there is no doubt that acetylcholine (ACh) functions as the major neurotransmitter that the medial olivocochlear neurons release onto the outer hair cells (OHCs) where it interacts with nicotinic receptors containing the $\alpha 9$ subunit to reduce the afferent output of the cochlea (see reviews: Bobbin, 1996, 1997; Bobbin & LeBlanc, 1999). Likewise there is no doubt that glutamate (Glu) functions as the primary neurotransmitter released by the inner hair cells to induce action potentials in the primary auditory nerve (Bledsoe, Bobbin, & Puel, 1988; Bobbin, Bledsoe, Winbery, & Jenison, 1985; Eybalin, 1993; Puel, 1995). In contrast, the neurotransmitter or neuromodulatory role of adenosine triphosphate (ATP) in the cochlea is yet to be completely defined (see reviews: Bobbin, 1996, 1997; Bobbin, Chen, Nenov, & Skellett, 1998; Housley, 1997). The role of ATP in the cochlea may be extensive because receptors for ATP appear to be on almost every cell in the cochlea. In various organ systems extracellular ATP has been suggested to serve as a neurotransmitter, neuromodulator, cytotoxin and mitogen (Burnstock, 1990; Dubyak & El-Moatassium, 1993; Fredholm, 1995; Wang, Huang, Heller, & Heppel, 1994; Zoeteweij, Van de Water, De Bont, & Nagelkerke, 1996). In the cochlea, ATP may act as: (1) a neuromodulator of cochlear mechanics (Bobbin et al., 1998; Chen, Skellett, Fallon, & Bobbin, 1998; Skellett, Chen, Fallon, Nenov, & Bobbin, 1997); (2) a regulator of potassium levels in the endolymph (Housley, 1997); (3) a mitogen, stimulating the proliferation of fibrocytes existing in the cochlea (Bobbin, Chu, Skellett, Campbell, & Fallon, 1997); and (4) a cytotoxin killing cells exposed to large amounts of ATP (Bobbin, et al., 1997). This chapter focuses on ATP and its role in the organ of Corti.

THE LOCATION OF ATP RECEPTORS IN THE COCHLEA

Both metabotropic (G protein mediated; P2Y) and ionotropic (P2X) ATP receptors may be present in the cochlea (Housley et al., 1999; Mockett, Bo, Housley, Thorne, & Burnstock, 1995; Xiang, Bo, & Burnstock, 1999). Definitive molecular biology evidence (mRNA levels) has been presented to show that the machinery for making P2X receptor protein is present in cells in the organ of Corti (Housley, Luo, & Ryan, 1998; Parker, Larroque, Campbell, Bobbin, & Deininger, 1998), spiral limbus, inner sulcus, spiral prominence and Reissner's membrane with low to undetectable levels in the stria vascularis (Housley et al., 1998). To date, a similar study has not been undertaken to describe the distribution of mRNA for P2YRs in the cochlea. However, there is physiological evidence for P2YRs in cells in the lateral wall of the cochlea (Ogawa & Schacht, 1995), marginal cells of the stria vascularis (Liu, Kozakura, & Marcus, 1995; Suzuki et al., 1995), in the organ of Corti (Niedzielski & Schacht, 1992) and in individual cells in the organ of Corti (e.g., **Deiters' cells:** Ashmore & Ohmori, 1990; Dulon, 1995; Dulon, Moataz, & Mollard, 1993; Moataz, Saito, & Dulon, 1992; **OHCs:** Ashmore & Ohmori, 1990; Ikeda, Saito, Nishiyama, Takasaka, 1991; Mammano et al., 1999; Nilles, Jarlebark, Zenner, & Heilbronn, 1994; **Hensen's cells:** Ashmore & Ohmori, 1990; Dulon et al., 1993; Sugasawa, Erostegui, Blanchet, & Dulon, 1996b; **IHCs:** Dulon, Mollard, & Aran, 1991; Sugasawa, Erostegui, Blanchet, & Dulon, 1996a; Yamashita, Amano, & Kumaawa, 1993; and **pillar cells:** Ashmore & Ohmori, 1990). In many cases, the physiological evidence was that application of ATP induced an increase in intracellular free calcium levels, which still occurred when extracellular calcium levels were reduced. From these studies the investigators concluded that the ATP receptors accounting for the increase in free calcium in the absence of extracellular calcium was P2Y receptors, which can release calcium from intracellular stores via a G protein mechanism (Ashmore & Ohmori, 1990; Dulon et al., 1993; Nilles et al., 1994 Sugasawa et al., 1996a, 1996b). There are other mechanisms that will explain the results. For instance, lowering extracellular calcium will not prevent ATP application from inducing an entrance of sodium into the cell via P2X receptors, which will result in a cellular depolarization. In skeletal muscle, for example, a depolarization can release calcium from intracellular stores without a G protein mechanism (Henzi & MacDermott, 1992; Rios & Brum, 1987). Thus the increase in intracellular calcium induced by ATP may not require the presence of P2Y receptors on the cells. Definitive evidence will be obtained with the demonstration in the cells of either the synthesis machinery (e.g., mRNA) or the protein for P2Y receptors.

Ionotropic responses to extracellular application of ATP presumably via $P2X_2$ ATP receptors have been recorded from several different cells isolated from the cochlea: (1) **outer hair cells** (OHCs; Ashmore & Ohmori, 1990; Chen, Nenov, & Bobbin, 1995; Chen, Nenov, Norris, & Bobbin, 1995, Chen, LeBlanc, & Bobbin, 1997, Chen et al., 1998; Housley, Greenwood, & Ashmore, 1992; Kakehata, Nakagawa, Takasaka, & Akaike, 1993; Kujawa, Erostegui, Fallon, Crist, & Bobbin, 1994; Lin, Hume, & Nuttall, 1993; Nakagawa, Akaike, Kimitsuki, Komune, & Arima, 1990; Skellett et al., 1997); (2) **inner hair cells** (IHCs; Sugasawa et al., 1996a); (3) **Deiters' cells:** Chen et al., 1998; Chen & Bobbin, 1998; Dulon, 1995; Skellett et al., 1997); (4) **Hensen's cells** (Sugasawa et al., 1996b); (5) **pillar cells** (Chen et al., 1998); and (6) **Reissner's membrane cells** (King, Housley, Raybould, Greenwood, & Salih, 1998).

As shown in Figure 6–1 various cells in the organ of Corti in the cochlea respond to the application of ATP with different shapes and forms of changes in cellular currents. These current responses apparently occur via the activation of P2X receptors on these cells. The OHCs of the guinea pig respond to ATP in an essentially nondesensitizing manner, maintaining ATP-induced current until the ATP is removed. In contrast, the supporting cells such as Deiters' and pillar cells respond with fairly rapid de-

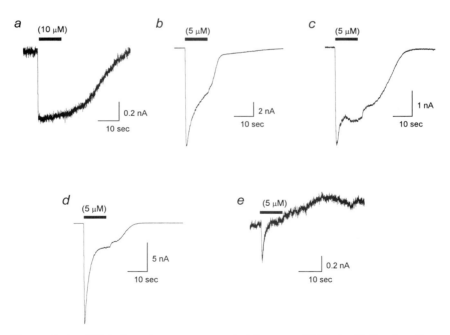

Figure 6–1. ATP-induced current recorded from **a**, OHC; **b**, Deiters' cell; **c**, Hensen's cell; **d**, pillar cell; and **e**, IHC; recorded in the whole cell voltage clamp mode (holding at −60 mV for OHC and IHC or at −80 mV for Deiters', Hensen's, and pillar cells). The concentration of ATP is given in parenthesis. For detailed methods see Chen et al. (1998).

sensitization where the current is greatly reduced almost immediately after the maximum current is produced. Hensen's cells and IHCs respond differently from OHCs and supporting cells. Such variations in phenotype between cells are thought to be due to differences in the subunit composition of the P2X receptors. Splicing of individual subunit mRNA and the expression of these different splice variants assembled into the receptors contributes to this variance in subunit composition of the receptors and their response to stimuli (e.g., Partin, Fleck, & Mayer, 1996).

TYPES OF P2X RECEPTORS IN THE COCHLEA IN THE ORGAN OF CORTI

Seven subunits of the P2X receptors (i.e., $P2X_1 - P2X_7$) and thirteen P2Y-like receptor protein sequences (i.e., $P2Y_{1-11}$, tp2y and fb1) have been isolated (Barnard, Simon, & Webb, 1997; King, Townsend-Nicholson, & Burnstock, 1998; North & Barnard, 1997). To date the $P2X_2$ subunit is the only receptor type mRNA that has been identified in the cochlea (Brandle et al., 1997; Chen & Bobbin, 1998; Housley, Greenwood, Bennett, & Ryan, 1995; Parker, Bobbin, & Deininger, 1997; Parker et al., 1998). In addition, several splice variants of ionotropic ATP receptors have been described (Brandle, et al., 1997; Housley et al., 1995; Koshimizu, Tomic, Van Goor, & Stojilkovic, 1998; Parker et al., 1997, 1998; Simon et al., 1997; Troyanovskaya & Wackym, 1998).

Since we and others have used the guinea pig as a test subject, it was important to discover the type of ATP receptors present in the guinea pig cochlea. Towards this end, we screened a guinea pig library kindly supplied to us by Wilcox and Fex (1992) for ATP receptors utilizing probes of rat sequences kindly supplied to us ($P2X_2$ by Brake, Wagenbach, & Julius, 1994). Utilizing this procedure we isolated and sequenced three clones. Two of the clones proved to be sequences that are very similar in sequence to two variants, $P2X_{2-1}$ and $P2X_{2-2}$, that have been isolated from rat tissue and so we have called them guinea pig $P2X_{2-1}$ and $P2X_{2-2}$ (Figure 6–2). The third is unusual in that it retained a "rat intron" that was spliced out of the rat sequence and so we have called it $P2X_{2-3}$ (Figure 6–2). To date such a splice variant has not been described elsewhere in the literature.

To determine the distribution of the three $P2X_2$ variants, and to see if the splice variant, $P2X_{2-3}$, was expressed in tissue other than in the cochlea, total RNA was obtained from guinea pig cerebellum, brain (cerebrum), kidney, liver, and testes as well as cochlea. Briefly, 50 mg of tissue (or two cochlea) were homogenized with TRIzol reagent (Life Technologies) and the RNA was extracted. RNA was separated by chloroform extraction, precipitated with isopropanol, washed in ethanol, and dissolved in DEPC-treated water. The RNA was treated with Dnase I (Life Technologies) to remove any contaminating chromosomal DNA. The cDNA was then synthesized from mRNA with oligo(dT)$_{12-18}$ primers using reverse tran-

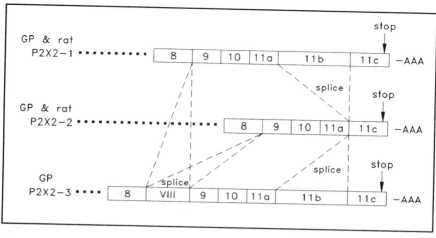

Figure 6–2. Organization of the guinea pig and rat P2X2 cDNA from exon 8 to the 3' end (poly A tail). The nucleotide sequence of rat and guinea pig variant P2X$_{2-1}$ cDNA is generated from exon 8 and 9 (intron VIII spliced out) and all of exon 11 (11a, 11b, and 11c). The nucleotide sequence of rat and guinea pig variant P2X$_{2-2}$ cDNA is generated from exon 8 and 9 (intron VIII spliced out) and a portion of exon 11 (11a and 11c; 11b spliced out). The nucleotide sequence of the guinea pig P2X$_{2-3}$ variant cDNA is generated from exon 8, intron VIII, exon 9, exon 10, and all of exon 11 (11a, 11b, and 11c). GenBank data base accession numbers are: AF053327 for P2X$_{2-1}$, AF053328 for P2X$_{2-2}$ and AF053329 for P2X$_{2-3}$. (From "Novel Variant of the P2X2 ATP Receptor From the Guinea Pig Organ of Corti," by M. S. Parker, M. L. Larroque, J. M. Campbell, R. P. Bobbin, & P. L. Deininger, 1998, p. 67. *Hearing Research, 121*, 62–70. Copyright 1998 by Hearing Research. Reprinted with permission.)

scriptase (Life Technologies). As a negative control, the reverse transcriptase enzyme was omitted from matching RNA samples ("no RT" control).

Nested PCR was carried out on first strand cDNA by first utilizing a set of primers that amplified DNA contained in both regions of interest, i.e., intron VIII and/or spliced putative exon 11. The outer primer set contained forward primer ttcacagagctggcacacag at nucleotide 785 and reverse primer aggaccagaagttcagagct at nucleotide 1541. PCR products from this reaction were subjected to a second round of PCR by utilizing an inner set of primers, which also amplified the regions of interest (nested PCR). The inner primer set contained forward primer tttggggtctgtgggtgtgg at nucleotide 856 and reverse primer tcatcccactgcaaccctaa nucleotide 1511.

PCR products were analyzed by 2% agarose gel electrophoresis. In addition to the "no RT" controls, negative controls included water instead of cDNA. Positive controls included PCR performed on plasmid DNA of each of the three guinea pig P2X variants (data not shown).

As seen in Figure 6–3A and 6–3B, the PCR amplification of cDNA from brain and cerebellum yielded strong P2X$_{2-2}$ (405 bp) and P2X$_{2-3}$ (675

Figure 6–3. A. Analysis of RT-PCR products by 2% agarose gel electrophoresis. Total RNA obtained from guinea pig cochlea, liver and testes was DNase treated, reverse transcribed, and the cDNA subjected to PCR using nested primer sets. Cochlea yielded strong P2X$_{2-2}$ (405 bp) and P2X$_{2-3}$ (675 bp) bands and also contained P2X$_{2-1}$ (594 bp). Liver yielded strong P2X$_{2-2}$ (405 bp) bands and also bands at 675 (P2X$_{2-3}$) and 594 (P2X$_{2-1}$). Testes yielded very strong P2X$_{2-2}$ (405 bp) and faint bands of P2X$_{2-3}$ (675 bp) and P2X$_{2-1}$ (594 bp). Identical reactions performed on cochlea RNA without reverse transcriptase were negative for PCR products. **B.** Analysis of RT-PCR products by 2% agarose gel electrophoresis. Total RNA obtained from guinea pig brain, cerebellum and kidney was DNase treated, reverse transcribed, and the cDNA subjected to PCR using nested primer sets. Brain and cerebellum yielded strong P2X$_{2-2}$

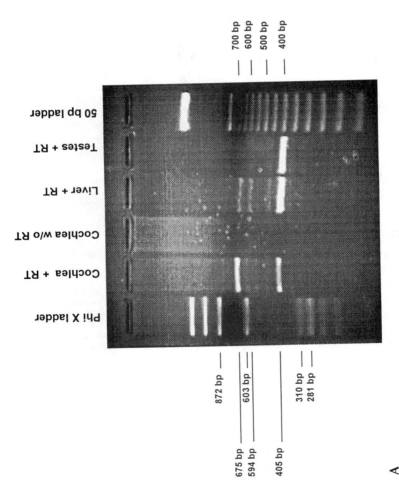

A

(405 bp) and $P2X_{2-3}$ (675 bp) bands and also contained $P2X_{2-1}$ (594 bp). Kidney yielded very strong $P2X_{2-2}$ (405 bp) bands and faint bands of $P2X_{2-3}$ (675 bp) and $P2X_{2-1}$ (594 bp). Nested PCR reactions with water replacing cDNA in PCR reactions was negative.

B

bp) bands and contained a moderate $P2X_{2-1}$ (594 bp) band. Kidney yielded a strong $P2X_{2-2}$ (405 bp) band and faint $P2X_{2-3}$ (675 bp) and $P2X_{2-1}$ (594 bp) bands . Liver yielded strong $P2X_{2-2}$ (405 bp) bands and faint $P2X_{2-3}$ (675 bp) and $P2X_{2-1}$ (594 bp) bands. Testes yielded strong $P2X_{2-2}$ (405 bp) and faint $P2X_{2-3}$ (675 bp) and $P2X_{2-1}$ (594 bp) bands. Cochlea yielded strong $P2X_{2-2}$ (405 bp) and $P2X_{2-3}$ (675 bp) bands and a faint $P2X_{2-1}$ (594 bp) band. Identical reactions performed on RNA from all the tissues without reverse transcriptase or with water replacing cDNA were negative for PCR products. In summary, the splice variant $P2X_{2-3}$ is strongly expressed in cochlea, brain, and cerebellum, and is weakly expressed in kidney, liver, and testes.

Presumably, the $3P2X_{2-3}$ splice variant found in guinea pig cannot be found in the rat. The reason is that the molecular mechanism that produces this variant in the guinea pig is the inclusion in guinea pig of a region analogous to rat intron VIII (Parker et al., 1998). The rat intron contains a stop codon. Therefore, even if the rat intron was expressed, presumably it would result in a truncated protein lacking the second transmembrane spanning region of the receptor.

This raises the question of why the guinea pig makes this splice variant and the rat does not and what effect this variant has on the function of the cochlea. To date there are only preliminary data on this question. Chen et al. (1997) failed to obtain responses to application of ATP in most rat outer hair cells. The exceptions were very small cells that were difficult to identify as OHCs and may not have been OHCs. In contrast these authors obtained large responses in guinea pig outer hair cells and in Deiters' cells from both rat and guinea pig. This suggests that the reason for the reduced incidence or absence of a response to ATP in rat OHCs may have been due to the absence of the $P2X_{2-3}$ splice variant in rat. It does appear that $P2X_2$ mRNA is present in rat outer hair cells (Housley et al., 1998) but the protein may not be expressed. Thus it will be interesting to look at the distribution of the $P2X_{2-3}$ splice variant and see if this subunit is present in guinea pig OHCs.

As shown in Figure 6–1, the OHC of guinea pig responds to the application of ATP with an inward current that is nondesensitizing. Thus the question arises as to whether the $P2X_{2-3}$ splice variant is nondesensitizing or imparts nondesensitizing characteristic to the expressed receptor. To examine this hypothesis, the three splice variants were individually and transiently expressed in human embryonic kidney cells (HEK293). The properties of the three $P2X_2$ receptor variants were characterized using the whole-cell voltage-clamp technique. The results indicate that the application of ATP induced inward currents in HEK293 cells expressing homomeric receptors containing each of the three splice variants in a dose-dependent manner (Figure 6–4). The ATP induced currents in HEK293 cells expressing $P2X_{2-1}$ and $P2X_{2-2}$ variants were large, about the same amplitude and desensitized rapidly. The responses had characteristics similar to

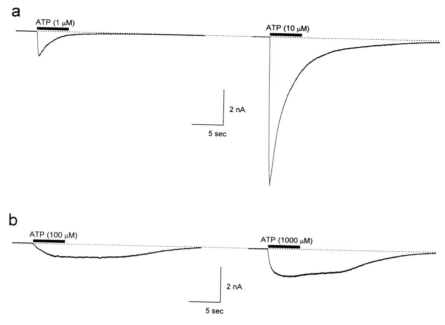

Figure 6–4. Current traces of ATP-induced responses recorded from transiently transfected HEK293 cells at a holding potential of −60 mV. **a.** Current traces for single cells expressing the $P2X_{2-2}$ splice variant in response to ATP application. **b.** Current traces for cells expressing the $P2X_{2-3}$ splice variant in response to ATP application.

those of the receptors on Deiters' cells in both rat and guinea pig (Chen et al., 1997; Chen & Bobbin, 1998). In comparison to the other two variants, the current in the cells expressing the $P2X_{2-3}$ variant was much smaller, required higher concentrations of ATP to be activated and desensitized slower. These results are consistent with the presence of the $P2X_{2-3}$ variant in OHCs partially accounting for the slow desensitizing response to ATP in OHCs compared to other cells in the organ of Corti. Since the guinea pig OHC response to ATP is a nondesensitizing response (Figure 6–1; Chen et al., 1997; Housley et al., 1992) and the $P2X_{2-3}$ splice variant is absent from the rat, then this variant is a good candidate for being the receptor present in guinea pig OHCs and the one absent from rat OHCs. This would indicate that the $P2X_{2-3}$ subunit may in part account for the nondesensitizing response in OHCs. Of course, there is a very high probability that additional splice variants, not described to date, exist in the organ of Corti. These undiscovered variants may be more important to the phenotype of the guinea pig OHC than the $P2X_{2-3}$ splice variant.

FUNCTION OF ATP AND ATP
RECEPTORS IN THE COCHLEA

ATP Receptors on Cell Surfaces Exposed to Endolymph

The ATP receptors on OHCs, Hensen's cells, IHCs, cells of Reisner's membrane, and cells in the stria have been suggested to be located on the cell surfaces exposed to endolymph rather than perilymph, although definitive location studies with antibodies for most of these cells remain to be carried out (OHCs: Housley et al., 1992; Mockett, Housley, & Thorne, 1994; IHCs: Sugasawa et al., 1996a; Hensen's cells: Sugasawa et al., 1996b; Reissner's: King, Housley, et al., 1998; stria: Liu et al., 1995). From this anatomical location of the various ATP receptors and physiological data obtained to date by various investigators, it appears that in general the ATP receptors bathed by endolymph are involved in cochlear fluid dynamics and movement of potassium across the cells lining the endolymph compartment (King, Housley, et al., 1998; Liu et al., 1995; Munoz, Thorne, Housley, & Billett, 1995; Munoz, Thorne, Housley, Billett, & Battersby, 1995; Suzuki et al., 1995). The ionotropic $P2X_2$ receptors on OHCs, which appear to be located on the steriocillia may be involved in transduction (Housley et al., 1992; Kirk & Yates, 1998; Mammano et al., 1999; Mockett et al., 1994, 1995). The origin of the endogenous ATP acting on these receptors may be the marginal cells of the stria vascularis (White et al., 1995).

ATP Receptors on Surfaces Lining the Perilymph Compartment

To date only Deiters' cells have been demonstrated to contain $P2X_2$ ionotropic ATP receptors exposed to perilymph (Dulon, 1995). These receptors appear to be located near where the Deiters' cell contacts the OHC (Dulon, 1995). Drugs placed in perilymph will act on these receptors exposed to perilymph, but not on receptors lining the endolymph compartment, due to cellular barriers that prevent drugs from entering endolymph from perilymph. Agonists that activate ATP receptors placed in perilymph decrease the magnitude of the cubic distortion product otoacoustic emissions (DPOAEs) and increase the magnitude of the quadratic DPOAEs (Figure 6–5; Kujawa, Erostegui, et al., 1994). The DPOAEs reflect the mechanical motion of the cochlear partition (Kemp, 1998; Mills, 1998). In addition, these agents alter cochlear sensitivity as monitored by changes in the summating potential (SP), the compound action potential of the auditory nerve (CAP), and N1 latency (Bobbin & Thompson, 1978; Kujawa, Erostegui, et al., 1994). Thus the tentative conclusion was reached that these drugs acted on $P2X_2$ ATP receptors exposed to perilymph or the ATP receptors on Deiters' cell (Bobbin et al., 1998).

Initially, the action of ATPR agonists (2-Me-S-ATP; ATP; ATP-γ-S) placed in perilymph was thought to be due to metabotropic, P2Y receptor

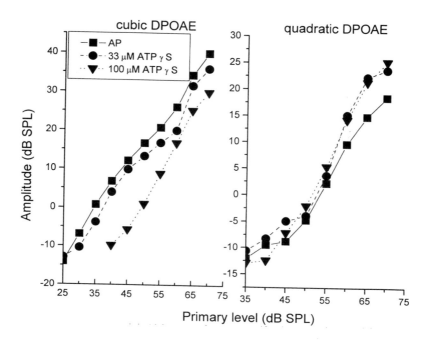

Figure 6–5. Dose response relationship of the suppression of the cubic DPOAE ($2f_1-f_2 = 8$ kHz; $f_2 = 12$ kHz) and enhancement of the quadratic DPOAE ($f_2-f_1 = 1.25$ kHz; $f_2 = 7.5$ kHz) induced by ATP-γ-S (100μM), an ATP receptors agonist. Shown are values obtained following perfusion of the perilymph compartment of the guinea pig for 15 min with a control perfusion (AP) and increasing concentrations of ATP-γ-S (33 & 100 μM). Data are represented as means ±S.E. across 2 animals.

activation (Kujawa, Erostegui, et al., 1994) as described by Niedzielski and Schacht (1992). However, 2-Me-S-ATP and ATP are rapidly broken down by ectonucleotidases, which exist in the perilymph compartment (Vlajkovic, Thorne, Munoz, & Housley, 1996). Due to this breakdown the in vivo potency of 2-Me-S-ATP and ATP at P2X receptors can be up to 1000 times less than that in vitro (Humphrey et al., 1995; Kennedy & Leff, 1995). In contrast, ATP-γ-S, which was the most potent compound in the Kujawa, Erostegui, et al. (1994) study is broken down very slowly. Confirming the notion that these drugs are rapidly degraded when placed in perilymph is the fact that, when applied to the isolated Deiters' cell, 2-Me-S-ATP is more effective than ATP (Chen & Bobbin, 1998) and at OHCs ATP is the same potency as ATP-γ-S (Kujawa, Erostegui, et al., 1994). In addition, ATP-γ-S is a powerful agonist at P2X receptors for which it has a very high affinity (Humphrey et al., 1995). Therefore, it appears that the action of these drugs in vivo may be due to the same $P2X_2$ receptors activated in vitro and not due to P2Y receptors as initially suggested by Kujawa, Erostegui, et al. (1994). On the other hand, at present there is no reason to eliminate an action of the drugs at P2Y ATP receptors and so one must be cautious in attributing the action of the drugs to either P2X or P2Y ATPRs until further studies are carried out.

Additional support for the Deiters' cell site-of-action hypothesis for the action of these drugs placed in perilymph are the observations of Dulon, Blanchet, and Laffon (1994). Dulon et al. (1994) demonstrated that Deiters' cells move and alter their tension in response to an increase in internal calcium levels. Since ATP induced activation of $P2X_2$ ATP receptors results in an inward current of Na^+ and Ca^{2+} in Deiters' cells (Figure 6–6; Ashmore & Ohmori, 1990; Dulon et al., 1993), ATP may also induce a stiff-

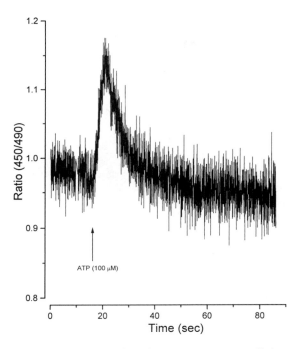

Figure 6–6. ATP-induced increase in intracellular Ca^{2+} in a Deiters' cell. Cell isolation and dye loading and measurements were carried out in the LSUMC calcium imaging facility utilizing a Noran's Odyssey laser scanning confocal microscope and data analysis software. Application of 100 µM ATP onto an indo-1/AM loaded Deiters' cell was by a pressure puff ejector via a glass pipette near the cell.

ness change in Deiters' cells. This change in stiffness may alter cochlear mechanics (Kolston & Ashmore, 1996) and be reflected as a change in DPOAEs (Figure 6–5; Kujawa, Erostegui, et al., 1994). At the apex of the cochlea, Deiters' cells hold the OHCs at their base and at their apical pole (Figure 6–7). In other turns of the cochlea, the Deiters' cell holds one OHC at the base and then an adjacent ones at the apical pole (see Figure 1–2 on page 13 in Brownell, 1996). An ATP-induced change in [Ca $^{2+}$] in Deiters' cells may alter the Deiters' cells tension, which in turn may act as a "bow" to tighten or loosen the tension on the string (OHCs). Since the shortening and lengthening of the OHCs appear to be responsible for the gain in the cochlear amplifier, then the alteration in stiffness of the Deiters' cells may act as a "set point adjustment" on the OHC motor to maintain an optimal gain. So the ATP agonists placed in perilymph and acting on P2X$_2$ ATP receptors on Deiters' cells may increase the stiffness of Deiters' cells to such an extent that the cochlear amplifier is unable to function and the cubic DPOAE is reduced and the quadratic enhanced (Figure. 6–5; Kujawa, Erostegui, et al., 1994).

MEASURES OF THE FUNCTION OF ENDOGENOUS ATP AND ATP RECEPTORS BATHED BY PERILYMPH

The Quadratic DPOAEs and SP

Frank and Kossl (1996) suggested that the quadratic DPOAE is a more sensitive indicator of the "set point" of the cochlear amplifier than the cubic DPOAE. van Emst (1996) suggested that the SP is also influenced by the "operating point of the apical transducer channel." The effects of suramin and PPADs, ATP antagonists, may be evidence that endogenous ATP affects the set point of the cochlear amplifier. Both drugs reversibly affect the quadratic DPOAE and suppressed the negative SP when the drugs were placed in the perilymph compartment (Chen et al., 1998; Kujawa, Fallon, et al., 1994; Skellett et al., 1997). PPADS (1 mM), which is much more potent than suramin in blocking the actions of ATP, induced more than a 10 dB suppression of the initial value of the time varying quadratic DPOAE (Chen et al., 1998). In addition, PPADS (1 mM) suppressed the quadratic DPOAE intensity function recorded immediately after a 15 min application of the drug in silence (Figure 6–8). This is in contrast to the little or no change in the intensity function of the quadratic DPOAE reported by Chen et al. (1998). This is explained by the fact that Chen et al. (1998) recorded the quadratic DPOAE intensity function 15 min after recording responses to the primaries, at which point the quadratic DPOAE had recovered to base line values. This indicates that these particular effects of PPADS on the quadratic DPOAE were readily reversible. In addition, PPADS had an

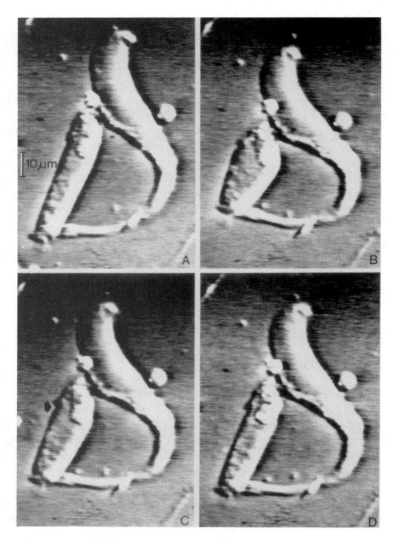

Figure 6–7. An example of an OHC being held by a Deiters' cell at the basal and api-cal pole of the OHC and the change in shape of the Deiters' cell as the OHC shortens and lengthens. Starting in the upper left frame (A) and following sequentially (B, C, D), the frames illustrate the change in shape of the complex during exposure to hypotonic saline. In frame B (upper right hand frame) the OHC has swollen and pulled on the Deiters' cell. This brings the phalangeal process of the Deiters' cell towards the Deit-ers' cell body. In frame C (lower left hand frame) the OHC has begun to burst (at the black arrow) and is expelling its contents and the OHC begins to lengthen returning the Deiters' cell towards the original point. In frame D (lower right hand frame) the OHC and the Deiters' cell have returned towards their original length. Note the Deit-ers' cell did not swell or burst in response to the hypotonic saline.

100

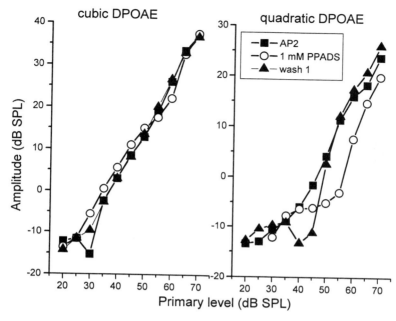

Figure 6–8. PPADS (1 mM) slightly enhances the growth functions for the cubic DPOAE ($2f_1 - f_2 = 8$ kHz; $f_2 = 12$ kHz) and suppresses the growth function for the quadratic DPOAE ($f_2 - f_1 = 1.25$ kHz; $f_2 = 7.5$ kHz). Shown are values obtained immediately following perfusion of the perilymph compartment in guinea pig with a control artificial perilymph perfusion (AP2), PPADS (1 mM) and a wash (wash 1). Perfusions were carried out in silence and recorded immediately after termination of the perfusion. The quadratic DPOAE values were collected first to avoid the reversal of the magnitude of the quadratic over time reported in Chen et al. (1998).

even larger effect (up to @20 dB sound equivalents) on the high intensity negative SP (scala vestibuli) that was readily reversible (Figure 6–9; Chen et al., 1998). These data are supportive of the speculation that these ATP receptor antagonists may induce their effects by blocking the depolarization and the increase in internal calcium in Deiters' cells induced by endogenous ATP acting on $P2X_2$ ATP receptors (Bobbin et al., 1998; Chen et al., 1998; Skellett et al., 1997).

Intense Sound Exposure

To further test the hypothesis that sound releases endogenous ATP to affect the function of the cochlea, the effect of PPADS on a moderately intense sound (95 dB SPL; 15 min; 6700 Hz) was tested. This level of sound

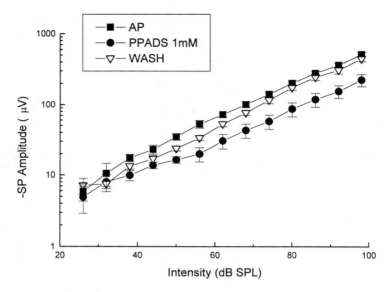

Figure 6–9. PPADS (1 mM) reversibly suppresses the negative SP recorded from scala vestibuli in response to 10 kHz tone bursts. Shown are the magnitude of the negative SP as a function of intensity recorded after predrug artificial perilymph perfusion (**AP**; 15 min), after perfusion with 1.0 mM PPADS (35 min), and after postdrug wash with artificial perilymph (**wash;** 15 min). All perfusions were through the perilymph compartment. Data are represented as means ± S.E. across 5 animals.

apparently induces only a temporary threshold shift as monitored by alterations in cochlear mechanics via DPOAEs (Puel, Bobbin, & Fallon, 1988). Therefore, it was reasoned that if endogenous ATP has an action on Deiters' cells to alter their stiffness then ATP may have a role in this sound-induced alteration in mechanics.

The methods used were very similar to those used previously (Puel et al., 1988; Puel, Ruel, d'Aldin, & Pujol, 1998). Animals were exposed to the pure tone 10 min after the start of a perfusion with artificial perilymph (intense sound group) or 1 mM PPADS (intense sound + PPADS group) and the tone was terminated 10 min before the end of perfusion. A third group received PPADs alone (PPADS alone group). Cochlear potentials evoked by 10 kHz tone bursts were recorded from an electrode in basal turn scala vestibuli. As shown in recordings of the cochlear microphonics (Figure 6–10) preliminary results indicate that the effects of the moderately intense sound combined with PPADS were larger than the effects induced by intense sound-alone or PPADS-alone. In addition, the enhanced effect was readily reversed with washing (Figure 6–10).

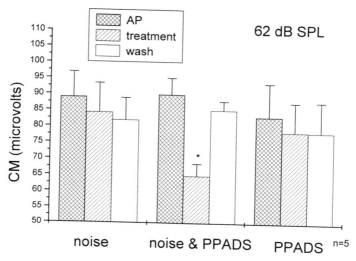

Figure 6–10. Effects of treatment with a moderately intense sound alone (**noise**, 6.7 kHz, 95 dB SPL, 15 min), a combination of the intense sound with 1 mM PPADs (**noise & ppads**) and 1 mM PPADS alone (**ppads**) on 62 dB SPL 10 kHz tone burst-evoked CM recorded from the scala vestibuli. Shown are values obtained after pretreatment artificial perilymph perfusion (AP), after treatment (i.e., noise exposure during AP perfusion; noise during ppads perfusion; ppads perfusion alone) and after washes with artificial perilymph (wash). The perilymph compartment was perfused. Data are displayed as means ± S.E. across $n = 5$ animals per treatment condition. The asterisk indicates a significant ($p < 0.05$) difference from AP and a significant ($p < 0.05$) difference from wash within treatment group.

These results are consistent with the hypothesis that endogenous extracellular ATP acting on ATP receptors on Deiters' cells increases the tension these cells apply to the motion of the OHCs and subsequently to the cochlear partition (Bobbin et al., 1998; Dulon, 1995; Dulon et al., 1993, 1994; Skellett et al., 1997). The PPADs block of these effects of endogenous ATP would indirectly decrease normal tension and so increase the motion induced by the moderately intense sound. This would in turn potentiate the effects of the intense sound.

There are many alternative explanations of these results and of the role of $P2X_2$ ATP receptors on Deiters' cells. Deiters' cells may play a role in the uptake and removal of extracellular K^+ that enters and exits the OHC as transduction current (Spicer, Smythe, & Schulte, 1999). An inward rectifying potassium channel is usually assigned this task; however, our laboratory has failed to find electrophysiological evidence for such a channel in Deiters' cells (Nenov, Chen, & Bobbin, 1998). Instead, extracellular ATP and the P2X$_2$ ATP receptors on Deiters' cells may be intimately involved in this removal of K$^+$. Activation of P2X$_2$ ATP receptors on Deiters' cells results in an increase in intracellular Ca^{2+} and Na$^+$ in a manner similar to the activation of excitatory amino acid receptors in glia (Gallo & Russell, 1995). By analogy with the relationship between neurons and glia (Gallo & Russell, 1995), this increase in Ca^{2+} and Na$^+$ could activate K$^+$ uptake through the efforts of a Na$^+$/Ca^{2+} exchanger and a Na$^+$/K$^+$ pump. In addition, if [Ca^{2+}] signals are propagated as a wave from the site of activity along the supporting cells coupled by gap junctions in a manner similar to glia, then the activation of P2X$_2$ ATP receptors may support spatial buffering of K$^+$ by drawing this ion away from the OHCs (as suggested for glia by Dietzel, Heinemann, & Lux, 1989; Gallo & Russell, 1995). Thus, during the moderately intense sound exposure in the presence of PPADS, there may have been an increase in extracellular K$^+$ concentration between the hair cells and the Deiters' cells due to a blockade of the K$^+$ uptake process involving P2X$_2$ ATP receptors in Deiters' cells. An increase in K$^+$ outside the basal end of the OHCs would produce a reduction in CM magnitude. Future experiments will determine if either or both the stiffness hypothesis and the K$^+$ hypothesis suggested here are correct.

The release of a chemical or neuromodulator onto these supporting cells in vivo during sound exposure was suggested by Oesterle and Dallos (1990) to explain the slow "end dc shift" they observed in electrical recordings from supporting cells during sound stimulation. Wangemann (1996) has shown release of ATP from an isolated whole organ of Corti into the fluid surrounding the tissue, presumably into the vicinity of the Deiters' cells. The source of the endogenous ATP acting on the ATP receptors on Deiters' cells may be the nerve endings forming synapses with these cells (Burgess, Adams, & Nadol, 1997).

SUMMARY

In summary, different cells in the cochlea exhibit different phenotypical responses to ATP. Preliminary evidence indicates that these phenotypes may be due to different combinations of P2X$_2$ splice variant subunits expressed in the different cells. In addition, it appears that extracellular ATP has several functions in the cochlea. One function in the endolymph compartment may be to regulate endolymph composition and the other function in the perilymph compartment may be to modulate cochlear mechanics or to ensure uptake of K$^+$.

Acknowledgments: This work was supported in part by a research grant from the National Science Foundation, American Hearing Research Foundation, the Deafness Research Foundation, the National Organization for Hearing Research, Kam's Fund for Hearing Research, the National Institutes of Health, and the Louisiana Lions Eye Foundation.

REFERENCES

Ashmore, J. F., & Ohmori, H. (1990). Control of intracellular calcium by ATP in isolated outer hair cells of the guinea-pig cochlea. *Journal of Physiology (London)*, *428*, 109–131.

Barnard, E. A., Simon, J., & Webb, T. E. (1997). Nucleotide receptors in the nervous system. *Molecular Neurobiology, 15*, 103–130.

Bledsoe, S. C., Jr., Bobbin, R. P., & Puel, J.-L. (1988). Neurotransmission in the inner ear. In A. F. Jahn & J. R. Santos-Sacchi (Eds.), *Physiology of hearing* (pp. 385–406). New York: Raven Press.

Bobbin, R. P. (1996). Chemical receptors on outer hair cells and their molecular mechanisms. In C. I. Berlin (Ed.), *Hair cells and hearing aids* (pp. 29–55). San Diego, CA: Singular Publishing Group.

Bobbin, R. P. (1997). Transmitters in the cochlea: The chemical machinery in the ear. In C. I. Berlin (Ed.), *Neurotransmission and hearing loss: Basic science, diagnosis, and management* (pp. 25–46). San Diego, CA: Singular Publishing Group.

Bobbin, R. P., Bledsoe, S. C., Jr., Winbery, S. L., & Jenison, G. L. (1985). Actions of putative neurotransmitters and other relevant compounds on *Xenopus* laevis lateral line. In D. G. Drescher (Ed.), *Auditory biochemistry* (pp. 102–122). Springfield, IL: Charles C. Thomas.

Bobbin, R. P., Chen, C., Nenov, A. P., & Skellett, R. A. (1998). Transmitters in the cochlea: The quadratic distortion product and its time varying response may reflect the function of ATP in the cochlea. In C. I. Berlin (Ed.), *Otoacoustic emissions* (pp. 61–83). San Diego, CA: Singular Publishing Group.

Bobbin, R. P., Chu, S., Skellett, R. A., Campbell, J., & Fallon, M. (1997). Cytotoxicity and mitogenicity of adenosine triphosphate in the cochlea. *Hearing Research, 113*, 155–164.

Bobbin, R. P., & LeBlanc, C. S. (1999). Apamin reduces but does not abolish the effects of contralateral suppression of cubic DPOAEs. In C. I. Berlin (Ed.), *The efferent auditory system* (pp. 61–71). San Diego, CA: Singular Publishing Group.

Bobbin, R. P., & Thompson, M. H. (1978). Effects of putative transmitters on afferent cochlear transmission. *Annals of Otology, Rhinology, and Laryngology, 87*, 185–190.

Brake, A. J., Wagenbach, M. J., & Julius, D. (1994). New structural motif for ligand-gated ion channels defined by an ionotropic ATP receptor. *Nature, 371*, 519–523.

Brandle, U., Spielmanns, P., Osteroth, R., Sim, J., Surprenant, A., Buell, G., Ruppersberg, J. P., Plinkert, P. K., Zenner, H. P., & Glowatzki, E. (1997). Desensitization of the P2X(2) receptor controlled by alternative splicing. *FEBS Letters, 404*, 294–298.

Brownell, W. E. (1996). Outer hair cell electromotility and otoacoustic emissions. In C. I. Berlin (Ed.), *Hair cells and hearing aids* (pp. 3–27). San Diego, CA: Singular Publishing Group.

Burgess, B. J., Adams, J. C., & Nadol, J. B., Jr. (1997). Morphologic evidence for innervation of Deiters' and Hensen's cells in the guinea pig. *Hearing Research, 108,* 74–82.

Burnstock, G. (1990). Purinergic mechanisms. In G. R. Dubyak & J. S. Fedan (Eds.), *Biological actions of extracellular ATP. Annals of the New York Academy of Science, 603,* 1–18.

Chen, C., & Bobbin, R. P. (1998). P2X receptors in cochlear Deiters' cells. *British Journal of Pharmacology, 124,* 337–344.

Chen, C., LeBlanc, C., & Bobbin, R. P. (1997). Differences in the distribution of responses to ATP and acetylcholine between outer hair cells of rat and guinea pig. *Hearing Research, 110,* 87–94.

Chen, C., Nenov, A., & Bobbin, R. P. (1995). Noise exposure alters the response of outer hair cells to ATP. *Hearing Research, 88,* 215–221.

Chen, C., Nenov, A. P., Norris, C., & Bobbin, R. P. (1995). ATP modulation of L-type Ca^{2+} channel currents in guinea pig outer hair cells. *Hearing Research, 86,* 25–33.

Chen, C., Skellett, R. A., Fallon, M., & Bobbin, R. P. (1998). Additional pharmacological evidence that endogenous ATP modulates cochlear mechanics. *Hearing Research, 118,* 47–61.

Dietzel, I., Heinemann, U., & Lux, H. D. (1989). Relations between slow extracellular potential changes, glial potassium buffering, and electrolyte and cellular volume changes during neuronal hyperactivity in cat brain. *Glia, 2,* 25–44.

Dubyak, G. R., & El-Moatassim, C. (1993). Signal transduction via P2-purinergic receptors for extracellular ATP and other nucleotides. *American Journal of Physiology, 265,* C577–C606.

Dulon, D. (1995). Ca^{2+} signaling in Deiters' cells of the guinea-pig cochlea active process in supporting cells? In A. Flock, D. Ottoson, & M. Ulfendahl (Eds.), *Active hearing* (pp. 195–207). London: Elsevier Science Ltd.

Dulon, D., Blanchet, C., & Laffon, E. (1994). Photo-released intracellular Ca^{2+} evokes reversible mechanical responses in supporting cells of the guinea-pig organ of Corti. *Biochemical and Biophysical Research Communications, 201,* 1263–1269.

Dulon, D. Moataz, R., & Mollard, P. (1993). Characterization of Ca^{2+} signals generated by extracellular nucleotides in supporting cells of the organ of Corti. *Cell Calcium 14,* 245– 254.

Dulon, D., Mollard, P., & Aran, J.-M. (1991). Extracellular ATP elevates cytosolic Ca^{2+} in cochlear inner hair cells. *NeuroReport 2,* 69–72.

Emst, M. G.,van (1996). *Origin of the cochlear summating potential in the guinea pig* [Thesis]. Department of Otorhinolaryngology, Utrecht University, Utrecht, Germany.

Eybalin, M. (1993). Neurotransmitters and neuromodulators of the mammalian cochlea. *Physiological Reviews, 73,* 309–373.

Frank, G., & Kossl, M. (1996). The acoustic two-tone distortions $2f_1-f_2$ and f_2-f_1 and their possible relation to changes in the operating point of the cochlear amplifier. *Hearing Research, 98,* 104–115.

Fredholm, B. B. (1995). Purinoceptors in the nervous system. *Pharmacology and Toxicology, 76,* 228–239.

Gallo, V., & Russell, J. T. (1995). Excitatory amino acid receptors in glia: Different subtypes for distinct functions. *Journal of Neuroscience Research, 42,* 1–8.

Henzi, V., & MacDermott, A. B. (1992). Characteristics and function of Ca^{2+}- and inositol 1,4,5-triphosphate-releasable stores of Ca^{2+} in neurons. *Neuroscience, 46,* 251–273.

Housley, G. D. (1997). Extracellular nucleotide signaling in the inner ear. *Molecular Neurobiology, 16*, 21–48.

Housley, G. D., Greenwood, D., & Ashmore, J. F. (1992). Localization of cholinergic and purinergic receptors on outer hair cells isolated from the guinea-pig cochlea. *Proceedings of the Royal Society of London, Series B: Biological Sciences (London), 249*, 265–273.

Housley, G. D., Greenwood, D., Bennett, T., & Ryan, A. F. (1995). Identification of a short form of the P2xR1-purinoceptor subunit produced by alternative splicing in the pituitary and cochlea. *Biochemical and Biophysical Research Communications, 212*, 501–508.

Housley, G. D., Kanjhan, R., Raybould, N. P., Greenwood, D., Salih, S. G., Jarlebark, L., Burton, L. D., Setz, V. C. M., Cannell, M. B., Soeller, C., Christie, D. L., Usami, S., Matsubara, A., Yoshie, H., Ryan, A. F., & Thorne, P. R. (1999). Expression of the $P2X_2$ receptor subunit of the ATP-gated ion channel in the cochlea: Implications for sound transduction and auditory neurotransmission. *Journal of Neuroscience, 19*, 8377–8388.

Housley, G. D., Luo, L., & Ryan, A. F. (1998). Localization of mRNA encoding the $P2X_2$ receptor subunit of the adenosine 5'-triphosphate-gated ion channel in the adult and developing rat inner ear by in situ hybridization. *Journal of Comparative Neurology, 393*, 403–414.

Humphrey, P. P. A., Buell, G., Kennedy, I., Khakh, B. S., Michel, A. D., Surprenant, A., & Trezise, D. J. (1995). New insights on P_{2X} purinoceptors. *Naunyn-Schmiedeberg's Archives of Pharmacology, 352*, 585–596.

Ikeda, K., Saito, Y., Nishiyama, A., & Takasaka, T. (1991). Effect of neuroregulators on the intracellular calcium level in the outer hair cell isolated from the guinea pig. *Otology, Rhinology, and Laryngology, 53*, 78–81.

Kakehata, S., Nakagawa, T., Takasaka, T., & Akaike, N. (1993). Cellular mechanism of acetylcholine-induced response in dissociated outer hair cells of guinea-pig cochlea. *Journal of Physiology (London), 463*, 227–244.

Kemp, D. T. (1998). Otoacoustic emissions: Distorted echos of the cochlea's traveling wave . In C. I. Berlin (Ed.), *Otoacoustic emissions: Basic science and clinical applications* (pp. 1–60). San Diego, CA: Singular Publishing Group.

Kennedy, C., & Leff, P. (1995). How should P_{2X} purinoceptors be classified pharmacologically? *Trends in Pharmacological Science, 16*, 168–174.

King, B. F., Townsend-Nicholson, A., & Burnstock, G. (1998). Metabotropic receptors for ATP and UTP: Exploring the correspondence between native and recombinant nucleotide receptors. *Trends in Pharmacological Science, 19*, 506–514.

King, M., Housley, G. D., Raybould, N. P., Greenwood, D., & Salih, S. G. (1998). Expression of ATP-gated ion channels by Reissner's membrane epithelial cells. *NeuroReport, 9*, 2467–2474.

Kirk, D. L., & Yates, G. K. (1998). ATP in endolymph enhances electrically evoked oto-acoustic emissions from the guinea pig cochlea. *Neuroscience Letters, 250*, 149–152.

Kolston, P. J., & Ashmore, J. F. (1996). Finite element micromechanical modeling of the cochlea in three dimensions. *Journal of the Acoustical Society of America, 99*, 455–467.

Koshimizu, T., Tomic, M., Van Goor, F., & Stojilkovic, S. S. (1998). Functional role of alternative splicing in pituitary $P2X_2$ receptor-channel activation and desensitization. *Molecular Endocrinology, 12*, 901–913.

Kujawa, S. G., Erostegui, C., Fallon, M., Crist, J., & Bobbin, R. P. (1994). Effects of Adenosine 5'-triphosphate and related agonists on cochlear function. *Hearing Research, 76,* 87–100.

Kujawa, S. G., Fallon, M., & Bobbin, R. P. (1994). ATP antagonists cibacron blue, basilen blue and suramin alter sound-evoked responses of the cochlea and auditory nerve. *Hearing Research, 78,* 181–188.

Lin, X, Hume, R. I., & Nuttall, A. L. (1993). Voltage-dependent block by neomycin of the ATP-induced whole cell current of guinea-pig outer hair cells. *Journal of Neurophysiology, 70,* 1593–1605.

Liu, J., Kozakura, K., & Marcus, D. (1995). Evidence for purinergic receptors in vestibular dark cell and strial marginal cell epithelia of the gerbil. *Auditory Neuroscience, 1,* 331–340.

Mammano, F., Frolenkov, G. I., Lagostena, L., Belyantseva, I. A., Kurc, M., Dodane, V., Colavita, A., & Kachar, B. (1999). ATP-induced Ca^{2+} release in cochlear outer hair cells: Localization of an inositol triphosphate-gated Ca^{2+} store to the base of the sensory hair bundle. *Journal of Neuroscience, 19,* 6918–6929.

Mills, D. M. (1998). Origin and implications of two "components" in distortion product otoacoustic emissions. In C. I. Berlin (Ed.), *Otoacoustic emissions: Basic science and clinical applications* (pp. 85–104). San Diego, CA: Singular Publishing Group.

Moataz, R., Saito, T., & Dulon, D. (1992). Evidence for voltage sensitive Ca^{2+} channels in supporting cells of the organ of Corti: Characterization by indo-1 fluorescence. *Advances in the Biosciences, 83,* 53–59.

Mockett, B. G., Bo, X., Housley, G. D., Thorne, P. R., & Burnstock, G. (1995). Autoradiographic labelling of P2 purinoceptors in the guinea pig cochlea. *Hearing Research, 84,* 177–193.

Mockett, B. G., Housley, G. D., & Thorne, P. R. (1994). Fluorescence imaging of extracellular purinergic receptor sites and putative ecto-ATPases sites on isolated cochlear hair cells. *Journal of Neuroscience, 14,* 6992–7007.

Munoz, D. J. B., Thorne, P. R., Housley, T. E., & Billett, T. E. (1995). Adenosine 5'-triphosphate (ATP) concentrations in the endolymph and perilymph of the guinea pig cochlea. *Hearing Research, 90,* 119–125.

Munoz, D. J. B., Thorne, P. R., Housley, T. E., Billett, T. E., & Battersby, J. M. (1995). Extracellular adenosine 5'-triphosphate (ATP) in the endolymphatic compartment influences cochlear function. *Hearing Research, 90,* 106–118.

Nakagawa, T., Akaike, N., Kimitsuki, T., Komune, S., & Arima, T. (1990). ATP-induced current in isolated outer hair cells of guinea pig cochlea. *Journal of Neurophysiology, 63,* 1068–1074.

Nenov, A. P., Chen, C., & Bobbin, R. P. (1998). Outward rectifying potassium currents are the dominant voltage activated currents present in Deiters' cells. *Hearing Research, 123,* 168–182.

Niedzielski, A. S., & Schacht, J. (1992). P_2 purinoceptors stimulate inositol phosphate release in the organ of Corti. *NeuroReport, 3,* 273–275.

Nilles, R., Jarlebark, L., Zenner, H. P., & Heilbronn, E. (1994). ATP-induced cytoplasmic $[Ca^{2+}]$ increases in isolated cochlear outer hair cells. Involved receptor and channel mechanisms. *Hearing Research, 73,* 27–34.

North, R. A., & Barnard, E. A. (1997). Nucleotide receptors. *Current Opinion in Neurobiology, 7,* 346–357.

Oesterle, E. C., & Dallos, P. (1990). Intracellular recordings from supporting cells in the guinea pig cochlea: DC potentials. *Journal of Neurophysiology, 64*, 617–636.

Ogawa, K., & Schacht, J. (1995). P2y purinergic receptors coupled to phosphoinositide hydrolysis in tissues of the cochlear lateral wall. *NeuroReport, 6*, 1538–1540.

Parker, M. S., Bobbin, R. P., & Deininger, P. L. (1997). Guinea pig organ of Corti contains mRNA for ATP receptor type P2X$_2$. *Association for Research in Otolaryngology Abstracts, 20*, 217.

Parker, M. S., Larroque, M. L., Campbell, J. M., Bobbin, R. P., & Deininger, P. L. (1998). Novel variant of the P2X$_2$ ATP receptor from the guinea pig organ of Corti. *Hearing Research, 121*, 62–70.

Partin, K. M., Fleck, M. W., & Mayer, M. L. (1996). AMPA receptor flip/flop mutants affecting deactivation, desensitization, and modulation by cyclothiazide, aniracetam, and thiocyanate. *Journal of Neuroscience, 16*, 6634–6647.

Puel, J. L. (1995). Chemical synaptic transmission in the cochlea. *Progress in Neurobiology, 47*, 449–476.

Puel, J. L., Bobbin, R. P., & Fallon, M. (1988). The active process is affected first by intense sound exposure. *Hearing Research, 37*, 53–64.

Puel, J. L., Ruel, J., d'Aldin, C. G., & Pujol, R. (1998). Excitotoxicity and repair of cochlear synapses after noise-trauma induced hearing loss. *NeuroReport, 9*, 2109–2114.

Rios, E., & Brum, G. (1987). Involvement of dihydropyridine receptors in excitation-contraction coupling in skeletal muscle. *Nature, 325*, 717–720.

Simon, J., Kidd, E. J., Smith, F. M., Chessell, I. P., Murrell-Lagnado, R., Humphrey, P. P. A., & Barnard, E. A. (1997). Localization and functional expression of splice variants of the P2X$_2$ receptor. *Molecular Pharmacology, 52*, 237–248.

Skellett, R. A., Chen, C., Fallon, M., Nenov, A. P., & Bobbin, R. P. (1997). Pharmacological evidence that endogenous ATP modulates cochlear mechanics. *Hearing Research, 111*, 42–54.

Spicer, S. S., Smythe, N., & Schulte, B. A. (1999). Distribution of canalicular reticulum in Deiters' cells and pillar cells of gerbil cochlea. *Hearing Research, 130*, 7–18.

Sugasawa, M., Erostegui, C., Blanchet, C., & Dulon, D. (1996a). ATP activates nonselective cation channels and calcium release in inner hair cells of the guinea pig cochlea. *Journal of Physiology (London), 491.3*, 707–718.

Sugasawa, M., Erostegui, C., Blanchet, C., & Dulon, D. (1996b). ATP activates a cation conductance and a Ca^{+2}-dependent Cl$^-$ conductance in Hensen cells of the guinea-pig cochlea. *American Journal of Physiology, 271*, C1817–1827.

Suzuki, M., Ikeda, K., Sunose, H., Hozawa, K., Kusakari, C., Katori, Y., & Takasaka, T. (1995). ATP-induced increase in intracellular Ca^{+2} concentration in the cultured marginal cell of the stria vascularis of guinea-pigs. *Hearing Research, 86*, 68–76.

Troyanovskaya, M., & Wackym, P. A. (1998). Evidence for three additional P2X$_2$ purinoceptor isoforms produced by alternative splicing in the adult rat vestibular end-organs. *Hearing Research, 126*, 201–209.

Vlajkovic, S. M., Thorne, P. R., Munoz, D. J. B., & Housley, G. D. (1996). Ectonucleotidase activity in the perilymphatic compartment of the guinea pig cochlea. *Hearing Research, 99*, 31–37.

Wang, D., Huang, N., Heller, E. J., & Heppel, L. A. (1994). A novel synergistic stimulation of Swiss 3T3 cells by extracellular ATP and mitogens with opposite effects on cAMP levels. *Journal of Biological Chemistry, 269*, 16648–16655.

Wangemann, P. (1996). Ca^{+2}-dependent release of ATP from the organ of Corti measured with a luciferin-luciferase bioluminescence assay. *Auditory Neuroscience, 2,* 187–192.

White, P. N., Thorne, P. R., Housley, G. D., Mockett, B., Billett, T. E., & Burnstock, G. (1995). Quinacrine staining of marginal cells in the stria vascularis of the guinea-pig cochlea: A possible source of extracellular ATP? *Hearing Research, 90,* 97–105.

Wilcox, E. R., & Fex, J. (1992). Construction of a cDNA library from microdissected guinea pig organ of Corti. *Hearing Research, 62,* 124–126.

Xiang, Z., Bo, X., & Burnstock, G. (1999). P2X receptor immunoreactivity in the rat cochlea, vestibular ganglion and cochlear nucleus. *Hearing Research, 128,* 190–196.

Yamashita, T., Amano, H., & Kumaawa, T. (1993). Efferent neurotransmitters and intracellular Ca^{+2} concentrations in inner hair cells of guinea pig. *Otology, Rhinology, and Laryngology, 55,* 201–204.

Zoeteweij, J. P., Van de Water, B., De Bont, H. J. G. M., & Nagelkerke, J. F., (1996). The role of a purinergic P_{2z} receptors in calcium-dependent cell killing of isolated rat hepatocytes by extracellular adenosine triphosphate. *Hepatology, 23,* 858–865.

Adaptation to Deafness in a Balinese Community

John T. Hinnant

Dr. Hinant did not present his work at the symposium, but it was so well represented by Dr. Friedman's comments, and the thought of learning more about this unique culture was so intriguing, that we invited Dr. Hinant to share his work and to share some videos of this fascinating work on the accompanying CD-ROM.

Communities have recently come to light in various parts of the world in which a fairly substantial deaf population has become integrated into the life of a larger populace. One of the most successful such adaptations occurred on Martha's Vineyard, Massachusetts in the 19th century (Groce, 1985). According to the memory of the oldest living inhabitants, a sign language known both to the deaf and the hearing citizens of the island enabled them to interact with apparent ease. Another such community is Providence Island, Colombia (Washtabaugh, 1980). In this case, also, the presence of a mutually intelligible sign language allowed a degree of interaction between deaf and hearing people. There are additional communities in Latin America, Africa, Nepal, and elsewhere in which a local sign language made possible both an interactive deaf community and accommodation to hearing people. Because communities in which successful accommodations to hearing loss are rare, each of these situations allows a special opportunity to understand the means by which hearing and deaf people can live together successfully.

Bengkala, Bali is another example of a successful accommodation of a deaf population to a community that has developed a unique sign language shared by deaf and hearing residents. The preceding chapter in this volume by Friedman et al., discussed the discovery of the community by two Indonesian physicians and the subsequent genetic research which has been carried out on the causative DFNB3 gene. This chapter provides a summary of the social and linguistic characteristics of the Bengkala deaf community.

111

THE VILLAGE OF BENGKALA, BALI

The village of Bengkala is located in the hill country of North Bali. As Friedman notes in the preceding chapter, *prasasti* (metal plates inscribed with proclamations from local kings, written in ancient Balinese script) associated with Bengkala are dated 1178 AD. They promulgate a legal code and set the geographical boundaries for a community that was apparently already flourishing and very much in need of regulation by the king of that time. Quite likely, the village antedates the arrival of Hindu religion on Bali.

Bengkala is a poor village. Because of its altitude, easily accessible groundwater is not available for the ubiquitous Balinese wet rice farming. Irrigation water, from Bali's famous *Subak* aqueduct system (Lansing, 1991), is only available for part of the village. Consequently, a variety of crops, centering on fruit production, are used to partially replace the vital rice crop as a source of food and income.

THE DEAF POPULATION OF BENGKALA

It is not possible to know exactly when the first deaf person was born in the village. Balinese Hindu ancestral beliefs cause a kind of genealogical amnesia (Geertz & Geertz, 1975). Two generations after a person has died, all memory of his name is lost. This makes good sense. In Balinese Hindu belief, each individual is reincarnated, and so a family's ancestors are now its children. There is no need to remember the ancestral names of individuals who are reincarnated. Not surprisingly, the first deaf person whose name appears on our genealogical charts has only been dead for two generations. Even if this person is not the first deaf individual, it is clear that there has been a steady increase, generation by generation, in the number of deaf people in the village. We have identified a total of 62 deaf individuals in the history of Bengkala, 48 of whom are still living. In families where deaf people have married deaf people, there are up to four generations of living deaf individuals present.

DEAF SOCIAL INTEGRATION IN BENGKALA

An understanding of the reasons Bengkala is one of the very few communities worldwide in which deaf people are well integrated into the social life of a community requires an excursion into the nature of Balinese Hindu society and into the organization of this particular village. Balinese villages are kin based. Groups of patrilineally related kinsmen live in residential clusters, or house yards. (Geertz & Geertz, 1975) In Bengkala, the deaf people live interspersed among their hearing relatives in several of the house yards. Consequently, the deaf grow up among a large number of hearing relatives. Small hearing and deaf children learn the unique sign language of the village together. Hearing children who grow up in this environment seem to learn sign language before they learn to speak. Signing is both part of communications and part of play. For the deaf children, exposure to the sign language occurs at birth. There is no part of their development in which they are deprived of the potential for symbolic communication. The crucial communicative contact between baby and mother is insured. Wherever a deaf baby looks, there is signing.

LIFE CYCLE AND SOCIAL IDENTITY

In discussing the lives of deaf people, it is perhaps best to start at the point which is, for us, the beginning—the birth of the baby. However, in Balinese Hindu religion, birth is merely one moment in a chain of births, deaths, and rebirths. Since babies are considered to be reincarnations of their ancestors, they are therefore sacred. For the first 6 months of their lives, their feet may not touch the profane earth. They must be carried everywhere by adults.

Reincarnation and Social Identity

When the baby is 1 month old, its father must go to a trance medium (*balian*) who contacts the ancestral realm to find out its former identity. Usually, the baby is identified as the reincarnation of one of its grandparents or of a dead relative from the grandparents' generation. On a few occasions, the trip to the trance medium can have genetic consequences. If, later in life, this baby-grown-to-adulthood has chronic misfortune, another trance medium may decide that the first medium was wrong. Instead of being the child of a particular family and the reincarnation of a particular ancestor, the individual in fact turns out to belong to an entirely different kin group. To remedy this situation, the individual must go through an identity change ritual, which involves a *wayang kulit* (leather puppet) performance. In Balinese conception, our world is a place of little importance. The realm of gods, temple spirits, and ancestors is the real world, which can only be seen through the screen of the puppet performance. (Lansing, 1983) The puppets impersonate divinities, and during the performances they reenact the lives of gods portrayed in the great Hindu sagas, the Mahabrata and Ramayana. The puppet master, the *Dalang*, is a man of enormous power, for it is he who mediates between this world and the world of the gods by controlling the actions of the puppets and speaking with all of their voices. During the puppet performance, through a particular puppet, the Dalang will indicate the new name and kinship affiliation of the distressed individual.

I have enough faith in Western empiricism to believe that the genetic material of the individual belongs to the first, culturally mistaken identity. During the process of preparing a comprehensive genealogy of Bengkala, I came across cases of individuals and their descendants being shifted entirely away from their biological parentage, and placed in the genealogies of other clans. For purposes of genetic analysis, we relocated them in their original kin groups. This instance is an example of the generally slippery nature of kinship systems, which are actually culturally determined and therefore variable. It also illustrates the fluid nature of personal identity in Bali.

The First Years of Life and Deafness

The general pattern of Balinese social maturation also applies to the deaf people. For 6 months, they are considered to be divinities whose feet must never touch the earth. Occasionally, during this 6-month period of very intense interaction with adults, it becomes apparent that a baby cannot hear. The infant is then subjected to sharp noises to see if it reacts. If the baby's parents are deaf, there is already the general expectation that the child will be deaf. Only in cases of hearing parents giving birth to deaf children is there any surprise.

There have been a number of situations in which a deaf baby is born to hearing parents who are heterozygotes for the recessive gene causing deafness in this community. The deaf members of the community, once they learn of such a child, visit and ensure that it learns to sign. Usually, the parents are already familiar with sign language and are able to teach the baby. However in 1998, a deaf baby was born to hearing parents who do not know the sign language. They are put in the awkward position of having to learn to sign as adults.

Maturation, Voluntary Groups, and Deaf Social Networks

As deaf children mature, they will join organizations that are peculiar to Balinese society. These organizations are called *sekeha*, and are voluntary groups that form around certain activities. When the activities are completed, the *sekeha* disband. There are *sekeha* for planting and harvesting rice. There are *sekeha* for a range of other agricultural tasks. There are even *sekeha* for making music and drinking palm wine. The financial goal of the *sekeha* in Bengkala is to save money to buy pigs for pork distribution at the festival of Galungan every 6 Balinese months. Additionally, for the deaf, the *sekeha* provide the opportunity to interact with hearing people in work situations that are not necessarily kinship based.

Deaf Exclusion From Age Grades and the Adat System

There is one area of the life of the village, a form of age grade organization, in which deaf people do not participate. The first grade, called *teruna/teruni* (for male/female members), begins when boys and girls are around the age of puberty. The young *teruna/teruni* form one of the most active groups in the village. They must always be present at temple ceremonies, and must carry out most of the work of preparing the Hindu temples for rituals. They also prepare secular celebrations. This organization is obviously an important means of socializing young adults.

The promotion out of this age grade occurs at marriage. Young men, who, through marriage, have recently become heads of households, join the *Desa Adat*. This is the council of household heads of the village. In Balinese villages, there are two systems of law. One is the traditional, or *Adat*, system and the other is the Indonesian legal system. Members of the *Desa Adat* regularly meet to discuss village issues, particularly issues concerning religious practice and the maintenance of the villages temples. Members of the *Adat* must contribute food and labor to major ceremonies, and they receive a special and highly prized ritual food called *lawar* in return.

Deaf children do not join the *teruna/teruni* system, and young deaf men do not join the *Desa Adat* at marriage. Issues that the deaf people wish to present at *Adat* meetings are voiced by a hearing member on their behalf; decisions reached by the *Adat* are signed to the deaf people after the meetings. Also, while the deaf do not contribute ingredients for the making of the all-important *lawar* at temple festivals, they do receive the same portion of the prepared ritual food as do members of the *Adat*.

Marriage

Throughout the fieldwork, issues centering around marriage, divorce, and domestic relations were the dominant topic of discourse. The deaf people marry at a fairly early age, even though finding a spouse is a difficult problem. Generally, deaf people marry one another, although there have been some deaf-hearing marriages. Several of the deaf have had a succession of spouses both hearing and deaf. Recently, some of the deaf people have begun to marry deaf people from other villages in hopes that children produced by these intervillage unions may not be deaf. Reciprocally, deaf men from other villages in the vicinity (in which there are very few deaf people) have begun visiting Bengkala in hopes of finding a wife.

Adult Life and Subsistence

The deaf people are farmers like the rest of the village community, and they inherit and use land like anyone else in the community. At present, many of the men are also employed as day laborers in the village and in other communities. Several of the women are seamstresses. According to oral history collected from the deaf and hearing members of the community, employment opportunities for the deaf have greatly improved in recent times. In the past, there was little wage labor, and what there was centered around water. As mentioned earlier, the village, with its high altitude, has a chronic water shortage. Deaf men received (very little) money from village households for carrying water in buckets from the river, which is located in a deep ravine at the edge of the village.

Today, there are two systems of piped-in water. The head of the village has continued the historical association between water and deaf people by placing them in charge of all of the water systems of the village. This involves continual effort and interaction with hearing people to keep the water pipes mended and operating. Deaf people are also in charge of water for temple ceremonies and festivals.

RELIGIOUS PARTICIPATION

There is an additional all embracing dimension of Balinese culture, its unique form of Hindu religion. It is with good reason that Margaret Mead in the 1940s wrote of the "the incredible busyness of the Balinese Hindus" (Bateson & Mead, 1942). On the village level, the Hinduism of Bali is a matter of continual ritual performance. Triggered by significant days in the island's ritual calendar, the more than 20,000 temples of Bali alternate in a continual cycle of elaborate celebration. Much of the effort of ritual preparation falls to women. Offerings, called *banten*, are constructed by women from flowers, banana and palm leaves, fruit, and cooked meat. Men are also involved in preparing *babi guling* (roast suckling pig) and other ritual essentials. Performances involve both sexes. Formal temple ceremonies require the recitation of mantras, which the deaf people do not know, but they do participate in the rest of the temple ceremonies. Women particularly are able to perform as well as their hearing friends in the preparation of ritual offerings.

There is a widespread belief in Bali that there are individuals capable of practicing magic, both good and bad. Other individuals, called *leyak*, are thought to be capable of transforming themselves at night into animals, traveling to people's homes, and mystically consuming their bodies over a course of many visits. In addition, there is a belief in *hantus*, the unquiet ghosts of those who have not been properly cremated. The deaf people are especially aware of this realm of beliefs. I have sat with them many evenings watching individuals sign stories of *leyaks* that they have seen and other extranormal events they claim to have witnessed. The evil doers are always hearing. This realm of belief seems to be more immediately real for the deaf people than are the mantra-based temple ceremonies.

SIGN LANGUAGE AND DEAFNESS

Indonesia has an official sign language, which is taught in schools for the deaf, but is not understood by the citizens of Bengkala. Bengkala sign language developed in the context of this one village and reflects the life of the village. It would be extremely difficult for an outsider to understand the language without having lived in the village with the deaf people.

Although there are many specific signs that can be applied in different contexts, much of the signing involves a complex narration of events (and gossip) using signs created specifically to communicate those events. The narration not only indicates what happens, but by the use of facial expressions and by body language, the whole feeling tone of the event is conveyed in ways more complete than mere speech allows. This narrational quality of the sign language poses a problem for a researcher from outside the village. By the end of each research trip, I have caught up on the narration of events and can usually understand what is being discussed. However, at the beginning of each new research trip, it becomes necessary to learn what has been happening lately and how it is represented in sign narration.

Bengkala sign has developed independently of writing. In Bali, there are many written languages—Indonesian, three Balinese languages, three Javanese languages, and Sanskrit. However, like many of the older hearing citizens of the village, the deaf people cannot read. Consequently, there is no finger spelling of unfamiliar terms. Also, the deaf do not know the names assigned them by their hearing relatives. Instead, they have an alternate system for identifying one another and their hearing compatriots. They use name signs. The unofficial leader of the deaf community has the privilege of assigning a name sign to each individual, deaf and hearing. The name signs are based either on some distinctive physical trait (a scar, a big nose in my case, and so on) or some aspect of character. These signs are not necessarily flattering or permanent. When some new and appealing aspect of an individual occurs to the deaf leader, he creates a new name sign and puts it into circulation.

Hearing loss is congenital. There is no evidence that the deaf people have ever heard sound. Tests, using a portable audiometer, were conducted with all of the deaf people. There was no evidence from the tests that anyone of any age was able to hear. The deaf, therefore, have no direct contact with spoken language. Their only contact with speech is possibly an indirect one. While the history of the development of the Bengkala sign language is not known, it seems reasonable to assume that hearing people were involved in its development. A question for future analysis is whether the grammatical structure of the sign language has parallels with the structure of spoken Balinese. My best guess at this point is that the sign language, like languages in general, has developed its own unique grammatical patterns.

Although the sign language centers on the use of hands, facial expressions, and body language, the deaf people are not silent when communicating. For example, an intensifier used to give emphasis involves making a popping sound with the lips. There are also sounds intended to attract the attention of hearing people. Each deaf person has his or her own distinctive attention getting sound. Also, some deaf individuals emphasize their general signing with a variety of vocalizations, especially during emotionally charged situations.

Although they are unable to hear in the usual sense, it is apparent that the deaf people are extremely sensitive to vibration. This first came to my attention when I was showing them a videotape I had made of them. At the same time, I was rewinding another videotape with a rather noisy rewinding machine. One of the deaf men turned around, puzzled, and seemed to be seeking the source of the sound. I showed him and then asked how he knew about it. He indicated that he felt it in his body. This sensitivity to vibration is particularly important for the involvement of some of the deaf people in a dance performance group.

MARTIAL ARTS AND DANCE

In the 1960s, two hearing men began independently teaching performance skills to a group of deaf men. The first of these hearing men was a gymnast and martial arts practitioner. Over a lengthy period of time he taught the complex and difficult sport called *pencak silat* to eight of the deaf men. They, in turned, instructed virtually the entire deaf community. Today, even the very small deaf children practice the sport.

The second hearing individual began the process of teaching classical Balinese dance to the same deaf men. In Bali, dance is a vital part of worship. It is believed that the Balinese gods periodically descend on each of the temples of Bali in turn expecting to be entertained with beautiful clothing, complex offerings, gamelan music, and dance. In any Balinese village, most people, male and female alike, have had some experience attempting classical Balinese dance. The instructor for the deaf dance group used a drum, rather than the usual gamelan orchestra, to provide the musical accompaniment for the dance. The deaf performers received their cues from the base vibration of the drum and the movement of the instructor's hands while drumming. Also, unknown to the audience at performances, the instructor signed instructions to the deaf performers between beats.

History of the Deaf Performance Group

The new found skills in both *silat* and dance were put to use when the eight deaf men formed a performance company under the direction of their hearing dance teacher. In the 1960s, this troupe traveled from village to village putting on performances before police groups (emphasizing *silat* combat) and in village settings (emphasizing dance performance). The troupe was well known. People from other villages have told me that they remember, as children, seeing the dancers from Bengkala perform. After being active for several years, the dance troupe disbanded because the hearing director and teacher became involved with commercial activities that demanded all of his time. The troupe was revived in the mid 1990s, after the Governor of Bali became interested in the deaf people. He assigned a professional dance teacher to prepare the troupe for public performances. While the original teacher had emphasized classical Balinese dance, the new instructor began lessons in dances of his own invention. He was apparently of the opinion that deafness is a great tragedy and that the deaf people are indeed sad. Several of his dances have them lamenting their deafness. He also taught them to perform using vocalizations. There are Balinese dances in which vocalizations are used but they are rare. Under this new teacher, a somewhat macabre, form of dance has recently emerged.

Both *silat* and dance skills have given the members of the deaf community a new series of options. *Silat* is used not only for personal defense and occasional performance, but also is the basis for membership by many of the deaf men and teenagers in the village guard, or *hancip*. Each evening, the *hancip* members, both hearing and deaf, gather and prepare to spend the evening sitting in the administrative offices at the center of the village. Occasionally they go out on patrol, but most of the time is spent exchanging stories and gossip. Sign language is used throughout, because almost always several of the deaf people participate in the rotating membership of the village guard. This interaction provides yet another situation for close communication between deaf and hearing people.

The Contemporary Importance of Performance

The combined *silat* and dance performances by the deaf people have put Bengkala on the media map. The deaf group has performed for both Balinese and national Indonesian television groups. Newspaper reporters have come to the village and have written about the deaf people. The deaf can see themselves occasionally performing on television. There is a plan for the deaf troupe to perform at the great Festival of Bali, which is held each summer for an international audience. All of this has created a real sense of accomplishment and recognition among the deaf community of Bengkala.

The finely honed skills required by *silat* and dance performance amply demonstrate that there do not seem to be significant vestibular problems in this deaf community in terms of body control. In some forms of deafness, individuals experience dizziness and other problems when attempting to carry out activities requiring a refined sense of balance. However, when a number of deaf and hearing people in Bengkala were specifically tested by asking them to close their eyes and walk in a straight line, the subjective state of several deaf individuals belied their obvious ability. They reported seeing stars behind their eyelids, dizziness, and a kind of drunken feeling. Many of the deaf people did not react in this manner, and none of the hearing people did so, including the hearing parents (obligate heterozygotes) of deaf individuals.

ATTITUDES ABOUT DEAFNESS

The word *kolok* is used to refer to the deaf. It refers to inability to speak, more than to inability to hear. It is a somewhat derogatory word, implying a lack of mental ability. It is generally used by people in the village who have little contact with the deaf people and little or no ability to sign. The kin, affines, and neighbors of deaf people generally refer to them by name or relationship, just as they would to anyone else in the community. They attach no stigma to deafness.

When asked about their own attitudes toward deafness, the deaf indicated that they want to hear. They believe their deafness limits their employment options. Several people, especially the teenagers, have signed their suspicion that hearing people laugh at them. Also, in a culture where music of many types fills the air, several of the deaf men and boys have lamented their inability to hear it. There is one exception. One young boy signed that he likes being deaf because it makes him special. Given the attention the deaf people have received from the Governor of Bali, the Indonesian media, and various visiting geneticists and anthropologists, his observation is reasonable. He intends to marry a deaf woman someday and wants to have deaf children. In 1998, he found an Indonesian sponsor who has taken him to Denpasar, the capital, where he has begun attending a school for the deaf.

DO THE DEAF HAVE A SEPARATE DEAF CULTURE?

One issue that should be discussed is whether there is a deaf community with a capital "D" having its own distinctive culture in Bengkala. The evidence is somewhat mixed. On several occasions, deaf people have told me how happy they are to leave behind the hearing members of the village, go out into the gardens, and simply be with one another. There they can sign much more quickly and do not have to worry about explaining the context of their signs to hearing people. There are many gatherings in the gardens for the purpose of feasting, drinking palm wine, practicing *silat* and other sports, and just gossiping about the hearing people. The deaf move about the village in one another's company and generally know more about one another's activities than they know about the activities of hearing people.

On the other hand, several of the deaf people, particularly women, do not participate in activities with the deaf community. They live at home and seldom appear with other deaf people. Also, when the deaf community throws a party in the gardens, inevitably a few of the particularly able signers among their hearing relatives are invited. Balinese people, hearing and deaf, are profoundly social. Connections among people based on kinship and marriage, along with membership in *sekeha* groups, temple groups, and so on, make it very difficult for any exclusive organization to exist among either the hearing or the deaf. The deaf people are immersed in the same complex social and cultural world as the hearing. They do not seem to have invented a distinct Deaf Culture that can be differentiated from that of the hearing. However, they have highly distinctive interests and experiences by virtue of deafness itself.

One thing is certain. Communication between the deaf and many hearing members of the community is continuous. There is a saying by the hearing community that the deaf people have no secrets. Since they communicate by signing and are forever signing with their hearing relatives and friends, events in their lives are widely known. Reciprocally, they care about the hearing people and are extraordinarily keen observers of their behavior and their foibles.

ONGOING RESEARCH

Since interdisciplinary research on deaf communities is a relatively new endeavor, it is perhaps useful to mention the types of social data that have been collected. To facilitate the genetic research, a comprehensive genealogy of the entire village of 2285 living individuals and more than 800 dead people, was constructed. At the same time a database was created with a record for each individual appearing in the genealogy. Using this information, we were able to connect 12 of the 13 kindreds originally collected by the two Indonesian physicians who discovered the village into one comprehensive picture of the deaf families. (See Figure 6–1 in the preceding chapter for an example of figures constructed from the geneologies.) The construction of accurate geneologies is probably the most useful thing an anthropologist can do for human genetic research. Because systems of kinship and marriage often have unpleasant surprises built into them as far as genetic research is concerned, it is also the job of the anthropologist to acquire a broad understanding of the culture and its impact on kinship and marriage. The instance of finding a new personal and kin identity mentioned earlier is one example.

In terms of the broader cultural and linguistic aspects of the research, I have so far spent almost 2 years living in the village with the deaf people, participating in events and watching what they do on a daily basis. This technique is called "participant observation" by anthropologists. It seems like no technique at all, but it is probably the most important one we have. In addition to daily observation, specific inquiries were made concerning the traditional history of the village and beliefs about the origin of its citizens. Medical beliefs were examined with a special emphasis on understanding the nature of deafness. The general economic and political life of the village was studied in order to evaluate the role of the deaf people. Extensive autobiographies of almost all of the deaf people were videotaped, and then laboriously translated from sign. Biographies of the deaf people were collected from many of their hearing neighbors and relatives. Nearly 100 hours of videotape and thousands of photographs (many taken by the deaf people themselves) were collected and will serve as one basis for further analysis of the language and social contexts of the deaf. And, of course, observation of the continual performance of Balinese Hindu rituals, and of those who participate in them, has been a backdrop for all other activities in the village.

CONCLUSION

A full account of the language and lives of the deaf people of Bengkala must await a book-length presentation, which is currently in preparation. As additional communities such as Bengkala are studied in detail, a clearer picture of the factors that differentiate between successful and unsuccessful social adaptations to profound deafness should emerge. Evidence from communities already studied suggests that a sign language known by deaf and hearing alike is vital. Social means for integrating deaf people into the larger community are also essential. In Bengkala, co-residence in kin-based house yards, obligations among kinsmen and affines, *sekeha* voluntary organization membership, civic responsibilities for water system maintenance and village guard duties, along with the endless cycle of religious events provide ample social integration of the deaf into the larger community.

Acknowledgments: None of this research would have been possible without the help of the deaf and hearing citizens of Bengkala. From the beginning, the deaf people have shared their language and their lives with us. While I was living in Bengkala, deaf people were either gathered in my host family's house yard, or I was in their houses or on some adventure in the gardens with them. Much of the still photography of the deaf people was the work of two of the technologically gifted deaf teenagers. Another major participant in the photography and in data gathering in general has been I. Ketut Kanta, my research assistant throughout the research. Since 1994, he has worked tirelessly year round keeping track of events in the lives of the deaf, including long periods when the demands of academic life kept me in America.

The two Indonesians who found the village, Drs. I. Nyoman Arhya and S. Winata, invited us to participate in the research, and facilitated the entire period of field investigation. Permission for fieldwork came from LIPI, the Indonesian Scientific Organization, and from the Governor of Bali. The members of the local Bengkala village administration provided hospitality and assistance throughout the fieldwork. Funding for the anthropological part of the research has been provided by the Deafness Research Foundation and by the Hearing Research Center at Michigan State University.

Final thanks go to Dr. Thomas Friedman who guided all aspects of the research, and who had faith that anthropology might be of benefit in investigations that usually are confined to the natural science disciplines related to genetics.

REFERENCES

Bateson, G., & Mead, M. (1942). *Balinese character, a photographic analysis.* New York: The New York Academy of Sciences.

Geertz, H., & Geertz, C. (1975). *Kinship in Bali.* Chicago: University of Chicago Press.

Groce, N. E. (1985). *Everyone here spoke sign language: Hereditary deafness on Martha's Vineyard.* Cambridge, MA: Harvard University Press.

Lansing, J. S. (1983). *The three worlds of Bali.* New York: Praeger.

Lansing, John Stephen (1991). *Priests and programmers: Technologies of power in the engineered landscape of Bali.* Princeton, NJ: Princeton University Press.

Washtabaugh, W. (1980). The organization and use of Providence Island sign language. In W. C. Stokoe (Ed.), *Sign language structure.* Silver Spring, MD: Linstok Press.

Appendix

Once we received the fascinating tapes from Dr. Hinnant on the Balinese sign language discussed in his chapter, we were content to leave that as the sole video on the CD-ROM that accompanies this book. However, when we played some of this material to colleagues in medicine and science, they all came back with the same question: **Is this the same sign language used all over the world?** It was not clear that sign languages differ around the world; American Sign Language differs from English Sign Language and French or Australian Sign Languages, although they are usually cross-interpretable with some effort.

We felt that a brief review and clarification of visual languages that are helpful to the Deaf was appropriate, and we decided to include examples of some of them. **Of the languages displayed, please keep in mind that ASL is *not* English on the hands; Cued Speech/Language, on the other hand, is a tool that puts any desired language on the hands for visual decoding.** This is not to imply that one is better than the other, just different, with different purposes and different histories

AMERICAN SIGN LANGUAGE OR ASL

ASL, the most common of the sign languages used in America, is described as the "Natural Language of the Deaf" by its proponents and is the *lingua franca* of the Culturally Deaf Community in America. Its presentation here in this book is owed to Ilene Miner, one of our highly respected colleagues who is a hearing social worker for the Deaf. Although her expertise is widespread, she is especially honored and respected for her work among patients and families with Usher syndrome. The segment here is part of an exchange between Ilene, a patient with Usher syndrome, and an audience of professionals many of whom were also Deaf.

The astute observer will note that the syntax and word order is not English on the hands (e.g., time is expressed spatially in front of the body for future occurrences and behind or over the shoulder for past occurrences) and that the hand movements, although highly descriptive, rarely carry phonologic information. The facial expressions and animation are especially noteworthy in Ilene's discourse. Note also that the interpreter sometimes loses her place and or "lags" since ASL is not interpretable word-for-word but needs to be creatively handled in "chunks". The visually impaired speaker was not aware of the problem and needed to be "tapped" to get her attention.

A great strength of ASL is its universal acceptance among the culturally Deaf, and its elegant and powerful linguistic structure. For those who doubt its legitimacy as a biologically based language, one need only read of its dependency on the same brain structures as in spoken language (see, for example, Hickock et al., 1999, *Brain and Language*, pp. 233–248; Hickock et al, 1996, *Nature*, pp. 699–702; and Corina et al., 1999, *Neuroimage*, pp. 570–581).

Its weaknesses involve the problems of hearing adults learning it as a second language in order to teach it to their Deaf children. It is a difficult language to learn (see Kemp, 1988, *American Annals of the Deaf*, pp 255–259). Late learners will almost always "have an accent" and will learn the language and its expression far better from a native Deaf person; in addition, it is reportedly quite difficult to teach native users of ASL to read and write English idiomatically, because they cannot "eavesdrop" on it. (See for example, Galvan, 1999, *American Annals of the Deaf*, pp. 320–324, or Fleetwood and Metzger, 1998, *Cued Language*.)

CUED LANGUAGE

(Originally Called Cued Speech)

Cued Speech was invented by Dr. Orin Cornett at Gallaudet University in a successful effort to make its practitioners literate in their native language. It uses four hand positions and eight hand shapes along with mouth positions to identify all the phonemes of English (and any other language for that matter) unambiguously. Its great strength is that it allows people who cannot hear to eavesdrop on the conversation of the users and absorb both language and culture; it does not require users to learn a new sign for each word or concept—just cue the phonemes in their own language.

Dr. Cathy Quenin supplied the excerpts on Cued Speech/Language from her dissertation. They show the effortless and virtually 100% accuracy of a deaf woman tracking a highly complex passage, in contrast to her having to lip-read and listen alone. Note especially the comfort and ease which the listener exhibits when cues are used, compared to the many errors and the frustration she experienced when lip-reading alone was required.

CODE SWITCHING FROM ASL TO
CUED LANGUAGE TO SPOKEN ENGLISH

As an added bonus, the CD-ROM includes an example of trilingual communication using spoken English, Cued Speech, and ASL. The scene is around a dining room table. In the center is a girl with a cochlear implant who is fluent in ASL. To her right is a deaf peer considering an implant. At the table is an adult male who also cues and is communicating with both girls. He cues to the girl in the center, she speaks back reasonably intelligibly and she communicates to the Deaf girl without speaking but using signs. In fact Cued Speech (better named Cued Language, see Fleetwood and Metzger, 1998) does not conflict with sign languages of any sort because they are so distinct, whereas various dialects of signs can and do conflict with one another.

Index

C

D

E

F